NTRA-ARTERIAL AND INTRACAVITARY CANCER CHEMOTHERAPY

DEVELOPMENTS IN ONCOLOGY

F.J. Cleton and J.W.I.M. Simons, eds., Genetic Origins of Tumour Cells
ISBN 90-247-2272-1
J. Aisner and P. Chang, eds., Cancer Treatment Research
ISBN 90-247-2358-2
B.W. Ongerboer de Visser, D.A. Bosch and W.M.H. van Woerkom-Eykenboom, eds., Neuro-oncology: Clinical and Experimental Aspects
ISBN 90-247-2421-X
K. Hellmann, P. Hilgard and S. Eccles, eds., Metastasis: Clinical and Experimental Aspects
ISBN 90-247-2424-4
H.F. Seigler, ed., Clinical Management of Melanoma
ISBN 90-247-2584-4
P. Correa and W. Haenszel, eds., Epidemiology of Cancer of the Digestive Tract
ISBN 90-247-2601-8
L.A. Liotta and I.R. Hart, eds., Tumour Invasion and Metastasis
ISBN 90-247-2611-5
J. Bánóczy, ed., Oral Leukoplakia
ISBN 90-247-2655-7
C. Tijssen, M. Halprin and L. Endtz, eds., Familial Brain Tumours
ISBN 90-247-2691-3
F.M. Muggia, C.W. Young and S.K. Carter, eds., Anthracycline Antibiotics in Cancer
ISBN 90-247-2711-1
B.W. Hancock, ed., Assessment of Tumour Response
ISBN 90-247-2712-X
D.E. Peterson, ed., Oral Complications of Cancer Chemotherapy
ISBN 0-89838-563-6
R. Mastrangelo, D.G. Poplack and R. Riccardi, eds., Central Nervous System Leukemia. Prevention and Treatment
ISBN 0-89838-570-9
A. Polliack, ed., Human Leukemias. Cytochemical and Ultrastructural Techniques in Diagnosis and Research
ISBN 0-89838-585-7
W. Davis, C. Maltoni and S. Tanneberger, eds., The Control of Tumor Growth and its Biological Bases
ISBN 0-89838-603-9
A.P.M. Heintz, C.Th. Griffiths and J.B. Trimbos, eds., Surgery in Gynecological Oncology
ISBN 0-89838-604-7
M.P. Hacker, E.B. Double and I. Krakoff, eds., Platinum Coordination Complexes in Cancer Chemotherapy
ISBN 0-89838-619-5
M.J. van Zwieten, The Rat as Animal Model in Breast Cancer Research: A Histopathological Study of Radiation- and Hormone-Induced Rat Mammary Tumors
ISBN 0-89838-624-1
B. Löwenberg and A. Hagenbeek, eds., Minimal Residual Disease in Acute Leukemia
ISBN 0-89838-630-6
C.J.H. van de Velde and P.H. Sugarbaker, eds., Liver Metastasis
ISBN 0-89838-648-5
D.J. Ruiter, K. Welvaart and S. Ferrone, eds., Cutaneous Melanoma and Precursor Lesions
ISBN 0-89838-689-6
S.B. Howell, ed., Intra-arterial and Intracavitary Cancer Chemotherapy
ISBN 0-89838-691-8

INTRA-ARTERIAL AND INTRACAVITARY CANCER CHEMOTHERAPY

Proceedings of the Conference on Intra-arterial and Intracavitary Chemotherapy, San Diego, California, February 24–25, 1984

edited by

Stephen B. HOWELL
Division of Hematology/Oncology
Department of Medicine
University of California, San Diego
School of Medicine
La Jolla, California, U.S.A.

1984 **MARTINUS NIJHOFF PUBLISHERS**
a member of the KLUWER ACADEMIC PUBLISHERS GROUP
BOSTON / DORDRECHT / LANCASTER

Distributors

for the United States and Canada: Kluwer Academic Publishers, 190 Old Derby Street, Hingham, MA 02043, USA
for the UK and Ireland: Kluwer Academic Publishers, MTP Press Limited, Falcon House, Queen Square, Lancaster LA1 1RN, England
for all other countries: Kluwer Academic Publishers Group, Distribution Center, P.O. Box 322, 3300 AH Dordrecht, The Netherlands

Library of Congress Catalogue Card Number 84-22615

ISBN 0-89838-691-8 (this volume)

PRINTED IN THE NETHERLANDS

INTRA-ARTERIAL AND INTRACAVITARY CHEMOTHERAPY

PREFACE

Both intra-arterial and intracavitary chemotherapy have been used for a long time. However, as is often the case, the clinical use of these regional techniques preceded the development of rigorous pharmacologic models, pharmacokinetic studies, and controlled clinical investigations. In most cases, the claims of therapeutic benefit were difficult to interpret or substantiate, and regional therapy attracted the attention of only a few dedicated physicians. The impetus for the symposium upon which this volume is based was that major advances in all three of these areas have been made in the past decade. Detailed pharmacokinetic models of both intra-arterial and intracavitary chemotherapy were developed that predicted substantial pharmacologic advantage to these routes of administration under certain circumstances. A number of careful pharmacokinetic studies have recently been published, and for the most part the results substantiate the predictions made from the models. We are now at a point where clinical trials based on these predictions are beginning to mature, and these make up the major component of the subject material covered in this symposium.

The field of regional chemotherapy is still in an early stage of development. The underlying hypothesis is that improving delivery of drug to the tumor will result in a greater tumor kill and a higher response rate. This hypothesis depends on the nature of the dose-response relationship for different kinds of tumors amenable to regional therapy. Whether these dose response curves are steep enough so that the increases in drug delivery achievable with regional therapy will be adequate to completely irradicate tumors not otherwise curable remains controversial. With the exception of intrathecal chemotherapy for meningeal malignancies, there is at this time insufficient data from controlled clinical trials to draw firm conclusions regarding therapeutic benefit.

This conference was organized with the aims of acquainting investigators with the pharmacologic rationale and technical aspects of delivering drugs by the intra-arterial and intracavitary routes, and updating clinical studies in those parts of the field that are moving rapidly. In addition, the last session of the conference focused on information from pre-clinical studies that is relevant to the design of new clinical investigations.

This conference was made possible through the generous support of many contributors. Among these, Adria Laboratories,Hoffmann-La Roche, Inc., and Pharmacia, Inc., deserve special mention. The support of all contributors is gratefully appreciated.

Stephen B. Howell, M.D.

TABLE OF CONTENTS

SESSION III: Clinical Trials of Intracavitary Chemotherapy

SESSION IV: Current Research on Novel Approaches

CONTRIBUTORS

KAREN H. ANTMAN, R. Osteen, and D. Montella, Harvard Medical School, Dana Farber Cancer Institute, 44 Binney Street, Boston, MA 02115

ROBERT M. BARONE, Department of Surgery, University of California, San Diego, 3930 Fourth Avenue, San Diego, CA 92103

JERRY M. COLLINS, Pharmacokinetic Section, Clinical Pharmacology Branch, Building 10, Room 6N 119, National Institute of Health, National Cancer Institute, Bethesda, MD 20205

FREDERICK R. EILBER, J. Mirra, J. Eckardt, and D. Kern, Division of Surgical Oncology, University of California, Los Angeles, 9th Floor Factor Building, 10833 Le Conte Avenue, Los Angeles, CA 90024

WILLIAM D. ENSMINGER, Internal Medicine and Pharmacology, Hematology and Oncology Division, University of Michigan, Ann Arbor, MI 48109

MARC B. GARNICK, B. Maxwell, R.S. Gibbs, and J.P. Richie, Sidney Farber Cancer Institute, 44 Binney Street, Boston, MA 02115

JOHN W. GYVES, Upjohn Center for Clinical Pharmacology, University of Michigan Medical Center, Ann Arbor, MI 40109

FRED H. HOCHBERG, A. Pruitt, D. Beck, G. DeBruyn, K. Davis, Harvard Medical School, Massachusetts General Hospital, Fruit Street, Boston, MA 02114

STEPHEN B. HOWELL, C.E. Pfeifle, and M. Markman, Cancer Center T-012, University of California, San Diego, La Jolla, CA 92093

STEPHEN C. JACOBS, Medical College of Wisconsin, 9200 West Wisconsin Avenue, Milwaukee, Wisconsin 53226

NANCY KEMENY, J. Daly, H. Chun, P. Oderman, G. Petroni, and N. Geller, Cornell University, Sloan-Kettering Hospital, 1275 York Avenue, New York, NY 10021

DANIEL E. LEHANE, Department of Pharmacology and Medicine, Baylor College of Medicine, 7580 Fannin Street, Suite 210, Houston, TX 77054

BRIAN J. LEWIS, R.J. Stagg, M.A. Friedman, R.J. Ignoffo, and D.C. Hohn, Cancer Research Institute, University of California,San Francisco, A-502, 400 Parnassus Avenue, San Francisco, CA 94143

WILLIAM E. LUCAS, Division of Reproductive Medicine, University of California, San Diego Medical Center, 225 W. Dickinson Street, San Diego, CA 92103

MAURIE MARKMAN, Cancer Center T-010, University of California, San Diego, La Jolla, CA 92093

STANLEY E. ORDER, Johns Hopkins Oncology Center, 601 N. Broadway, Baltimore, MD 21205

ROBERT F. OZOLS, R.C. Young, and C.E. Myers, Medical Branch, National Cancer Institute, 9000 Rockville Pike, Bethesda, MD 20205

YEHUDA Z. PATT, C. Charnsangavej, and M.Soski, Department of Medicine, University of Texas, M.D. Anderson Hospital, Houston, TX 77030

RALPH C. RICHARDSON[1], G.S. Elliott[1], J.M. Bartlett[1], W.E. Blevins[1], W. Janas[1], J.R. Hale[2], R.L. Silver[3], [1]Clinical Oncology, School of Veterinary Medicine, Purdue University, West Lafayette, Indiana 47907; [2]Francis Bitter National Magnet Laboratory, Massachusetts Institute of Technology, Cambridge, MA 02139; and [3]Michael Reese Hospital and Medical Center, Chicago, IL 60616.

F. KRISTIAN STORM, Division of Oncology, University of California, Los Angeles, Center for Health Sciences, 54-140, Los Angeles, CA 90024

THOMAS R. TRITTON[1], J.S. Lazo[1], P. Lane[1], D. Labaree[1], and L.B. Wingard, Jr.[2], [1]Department of Pharmacology, Yale Medical School, 333 Cedar Street, New Haven, CN 06510 and [2]Department of Pharmacology, University of Pittsburg School of Medicine, Pittsburg, PA 15261

SPONSORS

Adria Laboratories

Bristol-Myers Company

Cook Incorporated

Cormed Incorporated

Hoffman-La Roche Incorporated

Infusaid Corporation

Intermedic

Lederle Laboratories

Mead Johnson

Pharmacia

The Upjohn Company

'HARMACOKINETIC RATIONALE FOR INTRAARTERIAL THERAPY

'ERRY M. COLLINS

. INTRODUCTION

Now that a substantial number of anticancer drugs are ivailable, a high priority must be assigned to finding approaches 'hich will improve their use. EVERY anticancer drug has a narrow .herapeutic index, i.e., the dose which must be given for efficacy s a dose which is close to the maximum tolerated dose due to .oxicity.

The GOAL of intraarterial infusion is to increase the .herapeutic index, in other words, "to make a good drug better." 'here seem to be two opposing philosophies regarding intraarterial lrug delivery: some think it's so technically complex that it's ıever worthwhile, others get carried away by the alluring concept .hat if you deliver a drug directly to the tumor, it must be ıetter than intravenous delivery, regardless of the drug or the .ite. At this conference, I suspect that the first group is ınder-represented. The development of implantable pumps and other .echnical advances have made intraarterial infusions more widely .vailable, and the second group is expanding.

The role of pharmacokinetics and pharmacodynamics is not to :hoose sides, but rather to provide a quantitative perspective. hope to show WHY some drugs are attractive candidates for intra- .rterial infusion while others are duds, and also why some sites 'f delivery are more favorable than others (1,2,3,4). From a ractical standpoint, one quick calculation can save months and 'ears of clinical effort. Enthusiasm has a way of building. I ıave no intention of restraining it, but I'd like to encourage he enthusiasts to channel their resources into high-probability 'reas.

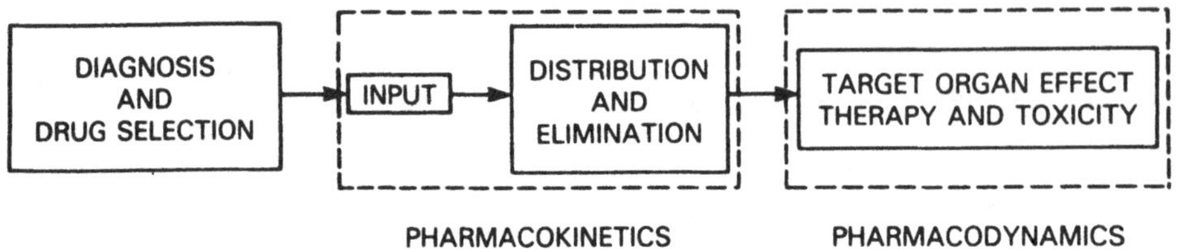

FIGURE 1. The distinction between pharmacokinetics and pharmacodynamics. From reference (4).

2. PHARMACODYNAMICS

As my title suggests, most of this presentation discusses pharmacokinetics. However, we must first clarify the distinction between drug kinetics and drug effects. As shown in Figure 1, pharmacokinetics is the description of drug concentrations during treatment, while pharmacodynamics is the description of drug effects, either therapeutic or toxic. The arrow which connects the two boxes indicates that there must be some relationship between these two domains, since the drug must reach its site of action or there will be no effect.

Our knowledge of pharmacodynamics is very primitive. In general, we would expect curves such as those shown in Figure 2 for response vs. concentration. As long as the maximum effect ha not been reached, increasing the drug concentration will increase the antitumor effect. However, host tissue toxicity will also be increased, which limits the maximum concentration that is tolerated. The goal of intraarterial therapy is to provide selective changes in concentrations: to increase tumor concentrations without raising the host tissue concentrations, and/or to decrease host tissue concentrations without lowering tumor concentrations.

As used in this presentation, the word "concentration" denotes the steady-state drug level achieved during a constant infusion. If "concentration" is interpreted as CxT, all formulas in this presentation are also valid for intermittent drug exposures. In the next two sections, it will be shown that it is possible to calculate the drug concentration ratio for

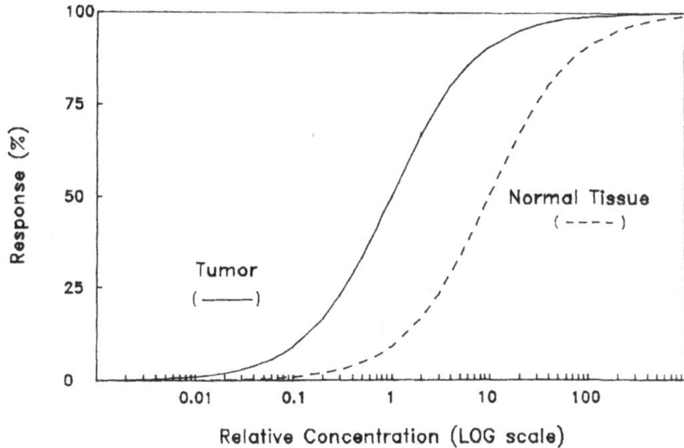

FIGURE 2. Response vs. concentration relationship for a typical drug. Solid line is for tumor, dashed line is for normal host tissue.

intraarterial vs. intravenous delivery. Both Figure 2 and these drug delivery ratios are limited to a description of total drug exposure. For anticancer drugs, time of exposure or threshold concentrations must often be considered in addition to total exposure.

The rest of my presentation will be restricted to pharmacokinetic considerations. I am assuming that the pharmacodynamics have been evaluated and that the goals of increased local concentrations and/or decreased systemic concentrations are reasonable.

3. INITIAL PHARMACOKINETIC CONSIDERATIONS

In the evaluation of the potential advantage of intraarterial infusions, the fundamental principle is that ALL of the advantage must result from the FIRST time the drug reaches its target. After the drug leaves the target and reaches the systemic circulation, it behaves the same as if it were delivered intravenously. The advantage of intraarterial administration should be assessed with reference to concentrations which are achievable by intravenous drug administration.

There are two ways that intraarterial infusion can increase the therapeutic index: (1) increase the concentration of drug achieved at the tumor site, and/or (2) decrease the concentratio of drug delivered to the rest of the body. The concentration in the rest of the body can only be decreased if there is local elimination of the infused drug before reaching the systemic circulation. This is referred to as the "first-pass" effect, and is primarily an issue for hepatic artery infusions.

Increased target concentration for intraarterial vs. intravenous delivery can be defined:

$$R_{target} = C_{target}(i.a.)/C_{target}(i.v.) \quad [1]$$

Similarly, the ratio of systemic drug exposures can be defined:

$$R_{systemic} = C_{systemic}(i.a.)/C_{systemic}(i.v.) \quad [2]$$

The overall advantage of intraarterial administration, R_d, is composed of the increased local concentration and/or the decreased systemic concentration:

$$R_d = \frac{R_{target}}{R_{systemic}} = \frac{C_{target}(i.a.)/C_{target}(i.v.)}{C_{systemic}(i.a.)/C_{systemic}(i.v.)} \quad [3]$$

Equation [3] is a general definition of the advantage of intraarterial delivery which is not dependent upon any particular pharmacokinetic model. It can be used to evaluate experimental results, but it has no predictive value. The following sections will develop formulas which can PREDICT R_d for various intraarterial situations.

4. INCREASED LOCAL CONCENTRATION (WITHOUT FIRST-PASS EFFECT)

Both conceptually and from the viewpoint of mathematics, it is easier to describe the case for which there is no first-pa effect. Figure 3 is a schematic representation of this case, using carotid artery infusion as an example. If there is no first-pass effect, then the systemic drug concentrations are identical (for the same dose, $R_{systemic}=1$). R_d is the ratio of target concentrations:

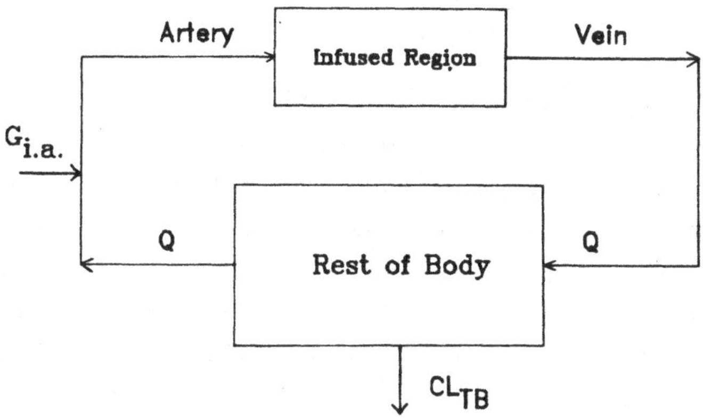

FIGURE 3. Schematic diagram for intraarterial infusion without a first-pass effect.

Table 1. Regional drug delivery advantage, R_d, for selected anticancer drugs. Based upon Equation [4].

CL_{TB} ml/min	Drug	R_d Q=100 ml/min	R_d Q=1000 ml/min
40000	Thymidine	401	41
25000	FUdR	251	26
4000	5-FU	41	5
3000	Ara-C	31	4
1000	BCNU	11	2
900	Adriamycin	10	1.9
400	AZQ	5	1.4
400	Cis-DDP	5	1.4
200	Methotrexate	3	1.2
--[a]	Cyclophosphamide	1	1

[a] Drugs which must be activated at a site other than the arterial infusion site have no drug delivery advantage.

$$R_d = \frac{C_{target}(i.a.)}{C_{target}(i.v.)} = 1 + \frac{CL_{TB}}{Q} \qquad [4]$$

CL_{TB} is total body clearance of the drug, which can be found in the literature or determined from intravenous doses. Q is blood flow in the infused artery, which can be estimated from physiology texts. For intraarterial infusions to most areas other than the liver, this is the only formula which is needed. The ratio of CL_{TB} to Q is the sole determinant of drug delivery advantage. This advantage can be calculated BEFORE doing an experiment or clinical study. Such calculations should influence the selection of drugs (based upon CL_{TB}) and sites of infusion (based upon Q).

R_d is calculated for various anticancer drugs in Table 1. A blood flow of 100 ml/min is used to illustrate a small artery and 1000 ml/min is used as an example of a large artery.

5. ROLE OF FIRST-PASS EFFECTS

5.1. Decreased Systemic Concentrations

If a certain fraction, E, of the infused dose is eliminated by the first-pass effect, then 1-E is available to the systemic circulation. For equal doses:

$$R_{systemic} = \frac{C_{systemic}(i.a.)}{C_{systemic}(i.v.)} = 1 - E \qquad [5]$$

If acute systemic toxicity is dose-limiting, a larger dose can be given intraarterially than intravenously. If cumulative systemic toxicity is dose-limiting, then a larger number of doses (or a longer infusion) can be given intraarterially.

5.2. Tumor Concentration

The first task is to determine if the first-pass effect occurs before or after tumor exposure. The most common situation for which this question is relevant is for tumor metastases to the liver. The critical determinant is the anatomy of the tumor blood supply, which is mostly determined by the size of the metastases.

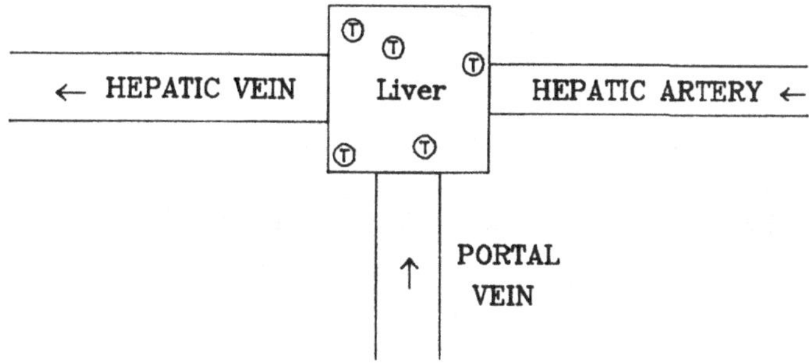

FIGURE 4. Blood supply to small hepatic metastases.

5.2.1 Small metastases. When the metastases are small, they are mingled with normal liver tissue (Figure 4) and derive their blood supply from the same sources as surrounding normal liver tissue (5). Regardless of whether the drug is delivered into th hepatic artery or the portal vein, it is effectively diluted by the TOTAL liver blood flow (Q_{HV}), since small metastases are nourished by both the heptatic artery and the portal vein:

$$R_{target} = \frac{C_{target}(i.a.)}{C_{target}(i.v.)} = 1 + \frac{CL_{body}}{Q_{HV}} \qquad [6]$$

Equation [6] is similar to Equation [4], except that total body clearance (CL_{TB}) has been replaced by CL_{body}, i.e., the clearanc in all areas of the body except the target area. Clearance with the target area (surrounding liver tissue) reduces the drug concentration delivered to the tumor for both i.v. and i.a. routes. R_d is calculated from Equation [6] divided by Equation [5]:

$$R_d = \frac{1 + \frac{CL_{body}}{Q_{HV}}}{(1-E)} \qquad [7]$$

If the liver is the only route of elimination (CL_{body}=0), the first-pass effect does NOT increase target concentrations:

$$R_{target} = \frac{C_{target}(i.a.)}{C_{target}(i.v.)} = 1 \qquad [8]$$

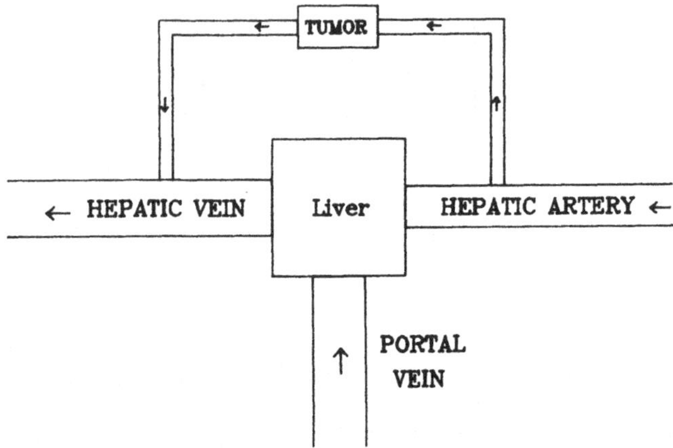

FIGURE 5. Blood supply to large hepatic metastases.

We should not conclude from Equation [8] that there is no advantage for intraarterial drug delivery in this circumstance. Systemic exposure will be lower as stated in Equation [5], and R_d will equal Equation [8] divided by Equation [5]:

$$R_d = \frac{1}{1 - E} \qquad [9]$$

5.2.2 Large metastases. As the hepatic metastases grow, they develop their own blood supply, chiefly from arterial vessels (5). As depicted in Figure 5, we can model large metastases as a separate compartment in parallel with normal liver. A fraction of the dose which is infused into the hepatic artery splits off to feed the tumor. Although larger metastases are usually a poor prognostic indicator, isolation of the blood supply from the degradative enzymes of normal liver tissue can enhance the therapeutic index. The effective tumor concentration can be higher than the concentration in normal liver tissue (or small metastases), since tumor tissue would not be expected to degrade the drug. This effect is not unique to intraarterial delivery but would also occur for intravenous administration.

The drug concentration in the tumor's branch of the hepatic artery should be the same as the drug concentration in the main branch of the hepatic artery. However, since the tumor cells are not nourished by the portal vein, the advantage of delivery via the hepatic artery is not diluted by the total liver blood flow:

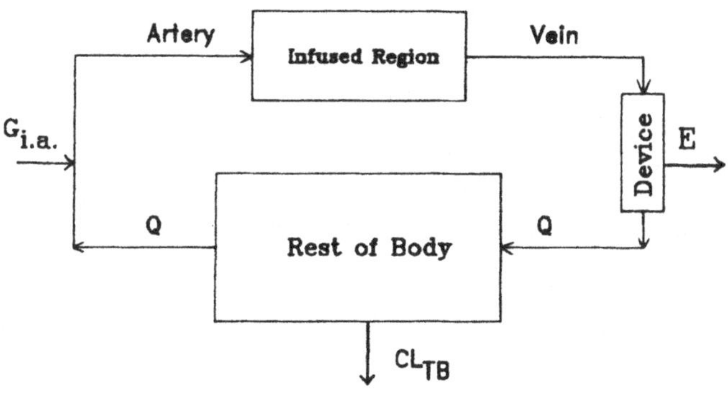

FIGURE 6. Schematic diagram of "extended" first-pass effect (6).

$$R_{target} = \frac{C_{target}(i.a.)}{C_{target}(i.v.)} = 1 + \frac{CL^*}{Q_{HA}} \qquad [10]$$

The value of the clearance parameter (CL*) lies between CL_{body} and CL_{TB}:

$$CL^* = CL_{body} + Q_{PoV}\, E \qquad [11]$$

Q_{PoV} is the portal vein blood flow.

The first-pass effect (1-E) is still present for systemic tissues. Therefore, the overall advantage is:

$$R_d = \frac{1 + \frac{CL^*}{Q_{HA}}}{(1-E)} \qquad [12]$$

5. EXTENDED FIRST-PASS EFFECT

For most drugs, the first-pass effect is normally limited to hepatic artery infusions. There is a collaborative project at NIH which attempts to overcome this limitation (6). This project involves the treatment of brain tumors with drug infusion into the carotid artery, followed by collection of jugular venous drainage and first-pass drug extraction by a hemoperfusion device before returning the blood to the systemic circulation. Schematically, this concept is shown in Figure 6. The modeling of this procedure yields a formula for R_d analogous to Equations [7] and [12]:

$$R_d = \frac{1 + \frac{CL_{TB}}{Q}}{(1-E)} \qquad [13]$$

Dr. Robert Dedrick is presenting a poster on this project at this Conference.

REFERENCES

1. Eckman WW, Patlak CS, Fenstermacher JD: A critical evaluation of the principles governing the advantages of intraarterial infusions. J. Pharmacokinet. Biopharm. 2:257-285,1974.
2. Chen HSG, Gross JF: Intra-arterial infusion of anticancer drugs: theoretic aspects of drug delivery and review of responses. Cancer Treat. Rep. 64:31-40, 1980.
3. Collins JM, Dedrick RL: Pharmacokinetics of Anticancer Drugs. In: Chabner BA (ed) Pharmacologic Principles of Cancer Treatment, W.B. Saunders, Philadelphia, 1982, pp 77-99.
4. Collins JM: Pharmacologic rationale for regional drug delivery. J. Clin. Oncol., in press, May 1984 issue.
5. Ensminger WD, Gyves JW: Regional cancer chemotherapy. Cancer Treat. Rep. 68:101-115, 1984.
6. Oldfield E, Dedrick RL, Chatterji DC, Yeager RL, Girton ME, Collins JM, Kornblith PL, Doppman JL: Reduced systemic drug exposure by combining intracarotid chemotherapy with hemoperfusion of jugular drainage. Surg. Forum 34:535-537, 1983.

TECHNICAL ASPECTS OF ARTERIAL ACCESS AND CONSTANT INFUSION

ROBERT M. BARONE, M.D. F.A.C.S.

Liver metastases are a common cause of death in colon carcinoma. One therapeutic modality for the treatment of these metastases for the past two decades has been direct hepatic artery drug infusion. However, this method has not gained popularity because of the difficulties encountered using external catheters and pumps needed to deliver this type of therapy. (1, 2, 3) Besides, of the reported intra-arterial results, none have proven statistically significant improvement in survival over intravenous 5-FU. There has been only one prospective randomized study reported comparing intra-arterial chemotherapy with systemic chemotherapy. (4) This study demonstrated no significant difference between systemic and intra-arterial chemotherapy. However, the intra-arterial chemotherapy was carried out for only a short period of time (three weeks), and all patients treated with intra-arterial chemotherapy subsequently received systemic chemotherapy. Recently, a number of investigators have reported response rates of 60 to 80 percent and improvement in median survival using the Infusaid* implantable infusion pump. (5,6,7) The system was first developed by Blackshear (8) at the University of Minnesota. From the preliminary reports using this system, it appears that the patients who will benefit most from this implantable system are those with colon metastases to liver only. (5,7) Other factors that play a role include the degree of liver involvement and histology. Selection of patients for this type of therapy should include the following work-up and criteria.

PREOPERATIVE EVALUATION

Preoperative work-up should include a chest x-ray, Technetium 99 Sulfur Colloid scan or computerized axial tomography of the liver to assess

---

* Infusaid Corporation - Norwood, Mass.

the degree of liver involvement. Either a liver scan, CT or ultrasound can be used for follow-up, depending on which one most clearly defines the lesions. An abdominal CT scan should be used to rule out extrahepatic disease, although this has proven to be of limited assistance in diagnosing small metastases on the peritoneum or small bowel. A Technetium 99 Sulfur Colloid scan is needed if the patient is found to have an abnormal blood supply to the liver and requires an intraoperative perfusion scan to ascertain perfusion. The Sulfur Colloid scan is needed for comparison with the intraoperative or postoperative scan to ascertain complete perfusion. Colonoscopy or barium enema may be needed for evaluation of the colon. Blood studies should include liver function tests, CBC, BUN, creatinine, prothrombin time and CEA. A bone scan need not be performed unless the patient is symptomatic or if one suspects sacral involvement from rectal carcinoma.

Contraindications to exploration and placement of a hepatic artery catheter include patients with severe malnutrition, a Karnofsky Performance Status of less than 60% (the patient requires considerable assistance and frequent medical care), portal systemic encephalopathy, malignant ascites, prolonged prothrombin time (with failure to correct with parenteral vitamin K to within three seconds of control), serum creatinine greater than 2.0 mg/dL, serum bilirubin greater than 4.0 mg/dL, serum albumin less than 2.5 g/dL or co-existent medical problems, such as pulmonary or cardiac disease, which would make the patient a poor surgical risk, or nephropathy, which may predispose to renal deterioration secondary to contrast agents during the preoperative work-up. Patients who have had radiation therapy to the porta hepatis are not good candidates since the porta hepatic tissues become quite fibrotic, making dissection of this area very difficult. This could result in injury to the common bile duct. In some instances where the patient has compromised liver function, one can treat the patient with a percutaneously placed catheter and intra-arterial chemotherapy for a period of time. If the liver function tests improve, then one can consider surgical exploration with placement of an implantable system at that time.

Once a patient is considered a candidate for intra-arterial therapy, the patient must then undergo preoperative assessment of the arterial blood supply to the liver. There are three major patterns of hepatic arterial anatomy. (9) The first, and most common, involves the right, middle and left hepatic artery arising from the hepatic artery off the celiac axis (Fig. 3). One major variation involves anomalous origin of the right hepatic artery from the superior mesenteric artery (Fig. 4). The other major variation is where the left hepatic artery arises from the left gastric artery (Fig. 5). The anomalous branches are either defined as accessory (representing additional supply to only a portion of a given lobe in addition to the normal blood supply usually off the celiac) or replaced (representing all of the blood supply to a given lobe). Even when an artery is accessory, it is possible that it is essential to the function of the hepatic segment which it supplies. Hepatic arteries are end arteries and, therefore, vital arterial contributors to the hepatic segments they supply.

The right lobe of the liver is supplied by the right hepatic artery. The lateral segment of the left lobe derives its supply from the left hepatic artery. The quadrate lobe (medial segment of the left) is primarily supplied by the middle hepatic artery, although small branches from the left hepatic artery often augment this. The blood supply from the quadrate lobe, in most cases, comes from the right hepatic artery, although in some instances the left or even middle hepatic arteries contribute.

After its origin from the celiac artery, the common hepatic artery runs along the upper border of the head of the pancreas forward and to the right, behind the posterior layer of the peritoneum of the omental bursa. At the level of the pyloroduodenal junction it courses anteriorly in the right hepatopancreatic fold. After running through the two layers of the lesser omentum and the hepatoduodenal ligament, it ascends to the liver with the bile duct lying to the right and the portal vein behind it. If either are replaced, or an accessory hepatic artery originates from the superior mesenteric artery behind the pancreas, it courses upward to the right and either behind or through the head of the pancreas before passing through the hepatopancreatic fold to the liver. Before its terminal distribution, the common hepatic artery usually gives rise to the gastroduodenal artery.

The right gastric artery arises from the common artery or left hepatic artery in about equal proportions (40%) and, less frequently, from the gastroduodenal artery (8%) or the middle or right hepatic artery (5%). It is usually small and difficult to find anatomically or angiographically. It descends to the pylorus, turns to the left and courses along the lesser curvature of the stomach where it anastomoses with the left gastric artery. It is best to ligate the tissue along the lesser curvature and distal one-third of the stomach in order to interrupt the blood supply to the stomach so as to prevent infusion of chemotherapy into the stomach.

The gastroduodenal artery usually arises from the common hepatic artery (75%). It may arise from the left hepatic (11%), right hepatic (7%) or superior mesenteric artery via the replaced hepatic trunk (3.5%). Sometimes it originates directly off the aorta, celiac axis or splenic artery. It descends behind the first portion of the duodenum anterior to the pancreas, courses to the left and, upon reaching the lower portion of the pancreas, it divides into the right gastroepiploic and the anterior superior pancreatoduodenal arteries.

The portion of the artery supplying the liver after the origin of the gastroduodenal artery from the common hepatic artery is named the hepatic artery proper. This portion of the hepatic artery ascends between the layers of the lesser omentum in the hepatoduodenal ligament. In most instances (85%) the right hepatic artery crosses the hepatic duct dorsally. Occasionally, the right hepatic artery is doubled, with one artery crossing the hepatic duct anteriorly and the other posteriorly. Usually, the right hepatic artery gives off 3 to 6 branches. One branch supplies the quadrate lobe while others enter the liver above the point of entry of the portal vein to supply the right lobe. When the right hepatic artery originates from the superior mesenteric artery, it passes behind the common duct and above and to the right of the portal vein.

The cystic artery typically arises to the right of the common duct from the right hepatic artery. In 20% it originates from the common hepatic, left hepatic, middle hepatic, gastroduodenal or retroduodenal artery, crossing the hepatic duct in most cases. In 25% the cystic artery is double.

In 75% of the cases, the left hepatic is a single artery arising most commonly from the hepatic artery proper. It enters the left lobe caudal to the left branch of the portal vein. In 25%, however, the entire left hepatic artery or an accessory left hepatic artery originates from the left gastric artery.

Of 157 consecutive angiograms performed for intra-arterial chemotherapy at Donald N. Sharp Memorial Community Hospital in San Diego, California, 87 (55%) demonstrated normal anatomy and 70 (45%) had abnormal anatomy.

The latter included 25 cases where the right hepatic originated from the superior mesenteric artery (Fig. 4); 16--left hepatic artery off the left gastric (Fig. 5); 2--trifurcation of right and left hepatic and gastroduodenal arteries off common hepatic (Fig. 6); 6--replaced common hepatic from superior mesenteric (Fig. 1-A); 9--reverse flow via gastroduodenal artery into proper hepatic artery (Fig. 1-B); 2--right hepatic from superior mesenteric with left hepatic originating from left gastric, middle hepatic and gastroduodenal off common hepatic (Fig. 1-C); 1--common hepatic artery arising as a common trunk above superior mesenteric artery, gastroduodenal artery off aorta, left gastric and splenic off celiac (Fig. 1-D); 1--independent origin of common hepatic off aorta below celiac with left gastric and splenic artery off celiac (Fig. 1-E); 1--replaced right hepatic off aorta above celiac artery with left hepatic and gastroduodenal arteries of common hepatic (Fig. 1-F); 1--right hepatic off superior mesenteric artery with left hepatic and gastroduodenal off aorta, left gastric and splenic off celiac (Fig. 1-G); 1--common hepatic with right and middle hepatic off celiac, gastroduodenal off celiac, left hepatic off left gastric.

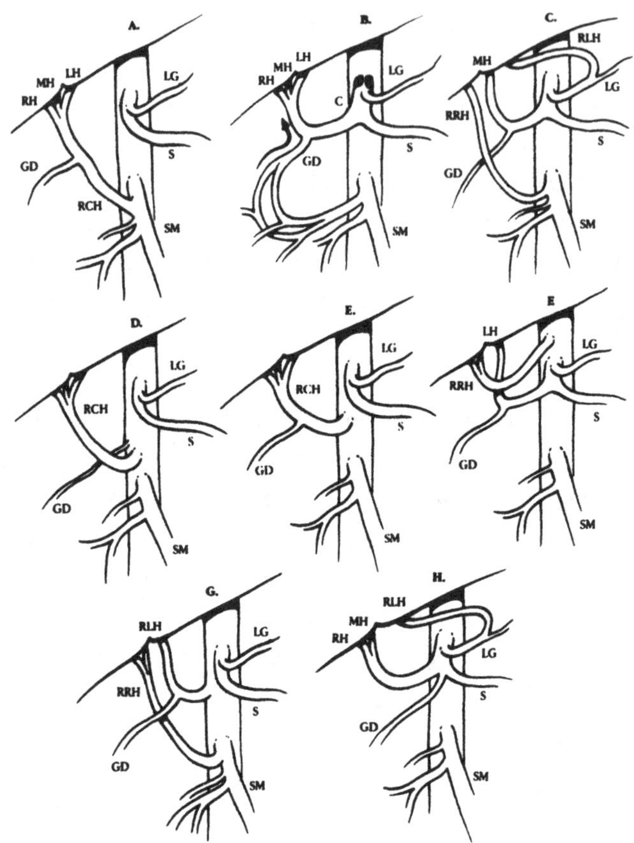

(FIGURE 1) VASCULAR VARIATIONS. RH - Right hepatic; MH - middle hepatic; LH - left hepatic; LG - left gastric; GD - gastroduodenal; S - splenic; RCH - replaced common hepatic; C - celiac; RRH - replaced right hepatic; RLH - replaced left hepatic.

1--Common hepatic off celiac, left hepatic off left gastric, gastroduodenal origin from splenic artery (Fig. 2-A); 1--early take-off of left hepatic off common hepatic (Fig. 2-B); 1--right and left hepatic with separate origin off celiac with gastroduodenal off left hepatic (Fig. 2-C); 1--common hepatic off left gastric, gastroduodenal off splenic artery (Fig. 2-D); 1--middle and left hepatic arteries off common hepatic, gastroduodenal off right hepatic (Fig. 2-E).

Other uncommon vascular anomalies have been described. (10) These include left hepatic arising from the superior mesenteric artery, common hepatic and gastroduodenal from celiac (Fig. 2-F); aberrant left hepatic artery arising from splenic artery (Fig. 2-G); replaced right hepatic from superior mesenteric, replaced left hepatic from left gastric with middle hepatic and gastroduodenal from celiac (Fig. 2-H); left hepatic arising from inferior phrenic (not pictured).

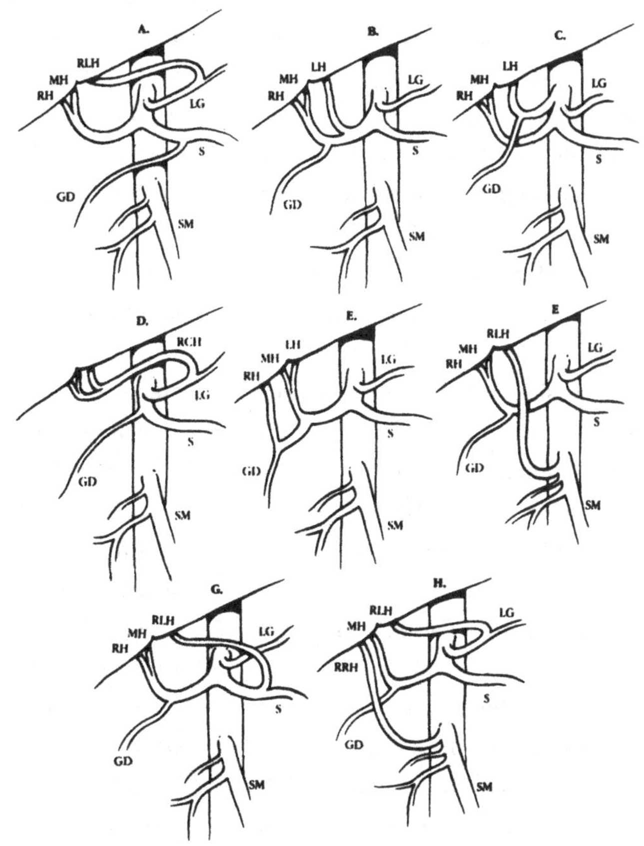

(FIGURE 2): VASCULAR VARIATIONS. RH - right hepatic; MH - middle hepatic; LH - left hepatic; LG - left gastric; GD - gastroduodenal; S - splenic; RCH - replaced common hepatic; C - celiac; RRH - replaced right hepatic; RLH - replaced left hepatic.

With an experienced invasive radiologist, most patients can undergo outpatient digital subtraction angiography preoperatively to determine vascular anatomy. In some cases, selective celiac and superior mesenteric angiography will be necessary to accurately define the vascular anatomy when digital subtraction angiography is unsuccessful in adequately determining the anatomy.

OPERATIVE PROCEDURES:

Only after the preoperative work-up is complete, and the vascular anatomy has been determined, is the patient taken to the operating room for surgery. The surgical procedure is performed through a midline incision and the abdomen thoroughly explored. If ascitic fluid is present, this should be sampled and sent for cytologic examination. Any suspicious nodules on the peritoneum, pelvis or serosa of the small or large bowel should be biopsied. A liver biopsy to document metastatic disease should be performed, as well as a needle biopsy of the uninvolved liver. In a few cases, underlying chronic hepatitis has been diagnosed. The patient may easily develop clinical hepatitis with minimal drug exposure. Notation of the location and size of the most prominent metastases and degree of liver involvement should be noted. The retroperitoneum should be palpated and any suspicious lymph nodes biopsied. Periportal, celiac and mesenteric lymph nodes should be inspected and palpated. Any suspicious lymph nodes should be biopsied. If the patient has significant extrahepatic disease, it is advisable not to implant the pump, since survival in this group of patients is poor.(5,7) One should consider placement of some type of portal in the face of extrahepatic disease. Only after it has been determined that one will be implanting a pump should it be removed from its sterile packaging and primed with Heparin and water. It is advisable not to fill the pump initially with chemotherapy. If the patient has an uneventful postoperative course, it can be filled with chemotherapy seven to fourteen days following surgery. Preparation of the implantable portals require no special care, but they should not be opened until one is sure they will be placed.

NORMAL ANATOMY (FIGURE 3)

Once the exploration and biopsies have been performed, the hepatogastric ligament superior to the pylorus is divided between clamps and ligated. One should avoid placing hemoclips in the region since it may interfere with catheter placement and later CT scanning. At times, hyperplastic lymph nodes are encountered in this location. It is helpful to remove these lymph nodes to facilitate exposure and also to rule out possible microscopic metastatic disease.

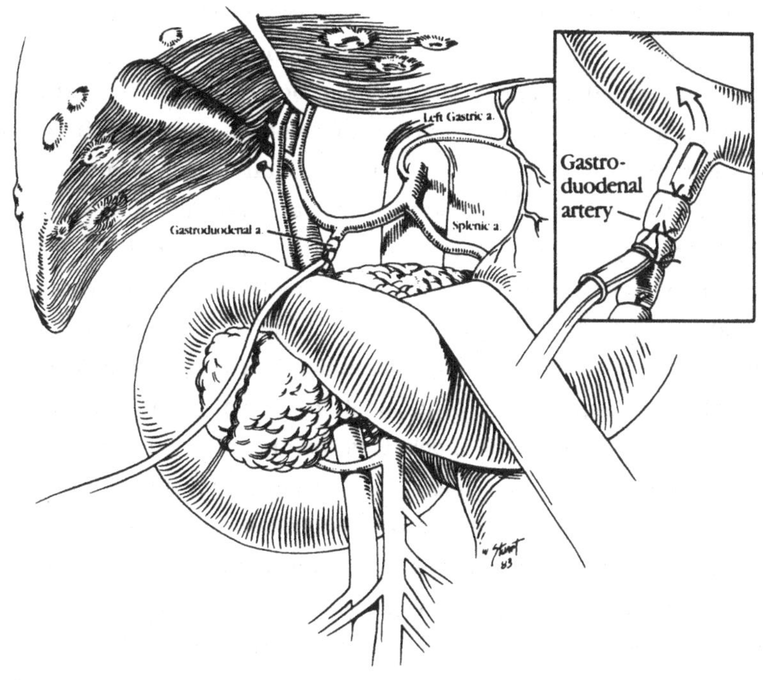

(FIGURE 3): CATHETER PLACEMENT NORMAL ANATOMY. Catheter placed through gastroduodenal artery into common hepatic artery.

Once the gastroduodenal artery is identified, it is skeletonized for 3 to 4 cm. The junction of the gastroduodenal artery origin from the common artery is identified, and the common hepatic - proper hepatic artery is skeletonized for several centimeters to attempty to identify the right gastric artery, which should be ligated. If it cannot be identified, the hepatoduodenal ligament should be divided along the lesser curvature from the pylorus to just below the incisura to interrupt the right gastric arterial supply to this area. This prevents drug infusion to this area and thus will prevent future duodenal and gastric ulceration caused by prolonged infusion of chemotherapy to this area. The proper hepatic artery should be skeletonized to identify the bifurcation of the right and left hepatic arteries. The location of the bifurcation to the gastroduodenal artery origin should be ascertained, and if it is less than 1 cm. from the bifurcation, one should then place the catheter via the splenic artery into the proximal common hepatic (Fig. 6).

Once the artery has been dissected, a pump pocket is fashioned above the rectus fascia through the midline incision or separate incisions in the right or left upper quadrant. One should be careful not to approximate the costal margin or iliac crest in order to prevent the pump from rubbing on these structures postoperatively. If a portal is to be used, a portal pocket should be made in the lower sternal area in the subcutaneous tissues. If primary colon resection is being carried out in conjunction with pump or portal placement, the pump should be placed first and the pump pocket fashioned through a separate incision in the right or left upper quadrant so that it does not communicate with the surgical incision. This will prevent pump pocket contamination if the patient should develop a wound infection. Once the pocket is fashioned, two medium hemovac catheters are placed into the pocket and secured to the skin. Drainage catheters are not needed if a portal is used. The pump or portal catheter is brought through the abdominal wall in the middle of the pump pocket, and the pump or portal placed into the pocket and secured to the rectus fascia or sternal fascia using two or three Prolene sutures. The hemovac catheters are placed above and below the pump and connected to suction. The gastroduodenal artery is ligated distally and a Satinsky or Derra vascular clamp placed across the gastroduodenal - common hepatic junction (Fig. 3) An anterior arteriotomy is made and enlarged using Pott scissors. The tip of the beaded silastic catheter is cut at a distance so that the tip of the catheter will lie just into the common hepatic artery. The catheter is secured in place using several #3-0 silk sutures proximal and distal to the bead, which sits at the proximal end of the arteriotomy. One should be sure that the most proximal tie on the gastroduodenal artery is beyond the proximal extent of the arteriotomy since bleeding can occur around the catheter. It is important not to thread the catheter into the proper hepatic artery or common hepatic artery since this may lead to thrombosis.

RIGHT HEPATIC OFF SUPERIOR MESENTERIC ARTERY (FIGURE 4)

As discussed previously, vascular anomalies are encountered quite often. In order to ensure total perfusion of the liver, it will be necessary to place catheters into positions other than the gastroduodenal artery. In patients who have a right hepatic artery originating from the superior mesenteric artery, the usual location of the right hepatic artery is posterior to the common duct and to the right and anterior and to the right of the portal vein. Although there appears to be a long length of artery on arteriogram, most of this artery lies within or beneath the pancreas, which makes it inaccessible. It is best to dissect out a 1½ to 2 cm. segment of the artery within the porta hepatis.

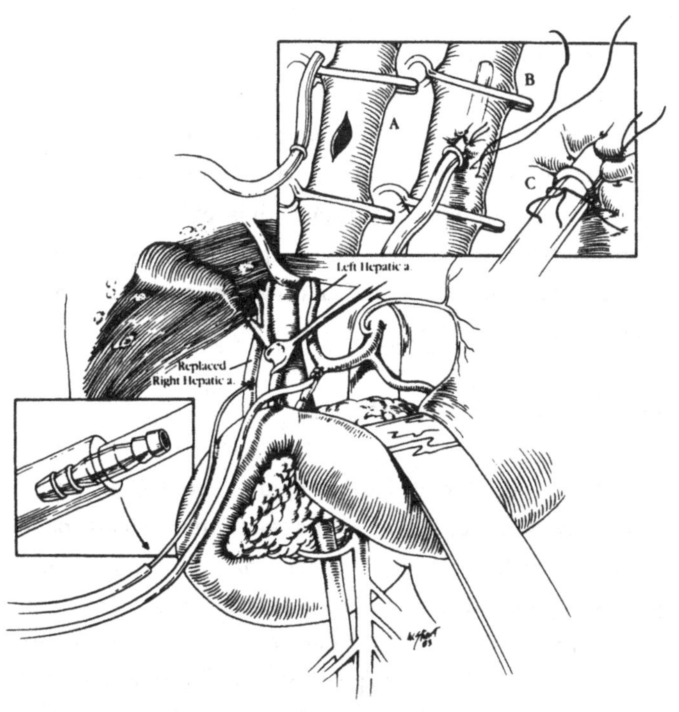

(FIGURE 4): CATHETER PLACEMENT FOR RIGHT HEPATIC OFF SUPERIOR MESENTERIC ARTERY AND LEFT HEPATIC OFF CELIAC. Catheter placed end to side into right hepatic. Inserts demonstrate connections between catheters and technique of securing catheter.

There are no side branches through which one could place a catheter. Therefore, it is necessary to place the catheter directly into the artery. Since the pump or portal catheter has an outside diameter of 2.3 mm., it is too large to place directly into the right hepatic artery. A silastic catheter measuring 4 to 6 inches in length with an outside diameter of 0.065 inches (Dow-Corning) can be fashioned. A 2 mm. segment of the tip of the catheter can be cut off and, using a straight mosquito, placed into the lumen of this cut segment. It is then placed over the tip of the catheter $1\frac{1}{2}$ to 2 cm. from the tip in similar fashion as the bead on the end of the pump catheter. Using McFadden aneurysm clips, a 1 to $1\frac{1}{2}$ cm. segment of artery is isolated (Insert Fig. 4). An anterior arteriotomy is made using a #11 blade. The catheter is placed into the hepatic artery up to the silastic ring. Using #6-0 Prolene suture, a pursestring is placed through the adventitia and tied. The tails of the Prolene suture are then tied above the ring around the catheter to secure the catheter into the artery. Loop magnification is sometimes helpful in placing and securing this catheter. This catheter is then connected to the pump catheter or portal using a connector.* The side port of the pump is flushed using heparinized saline to rule out subintimal dissection. A second catheter connected to an implantable device (Infusaport, Port-a-Cath, or Cormed) can be placed into the gastroduodenal artery using the technique shown in figure 3 to perfuse the left lobe.

INTRAOPERATIVE PERFUSION SCAN

Ligation of a replaced or accessory hepatic artery can be performed in some instances. However, one should be cautioned about performing this routinely. If one is considering placement of one catheter and ligation of the accessory vessel, an intraoperative Technetium 99 MAA perfusion scan should be performed. (11) One needs to have a portable gamma scintillation camera interfaced to a portable microcomputer brought to the operating room. The vascular supply is isolated and the catheter placed into the dominant artery. The accessory or aberrant artery is temporarily occluded using a vascular clamp or a McFadden aneurysm clip. Two to four millicuries of Technetium 99 macroaggregated albumin are injected through the catheter placed into the artery and flushed with heparinized saline after the gamma camera is positioned over the liver. Preoperative Technetium 99 Sulfur Colloid liver scan should be available

---

* Infusaid Corporation, Norwood, Mass. Part #35614-B

for comparison. If there is complete perfusion, then one can ligate the accessory replaced artery after comparison with the Sulfur Colloid liver scan. If it appears that a significant amount of the liver is not perfused, then one will need to place a second catheter. There is now available an infusion pump with two catheters which would allow perfusion to both lobes. If this is unavailable, then a second catheter and portal will need to be placed into the accessory or aberrant artery. A perfusion scan should then be performed through this second catheter to make sure that the accessory lobe is being perfused. Postoperatively an external pumping device such as Cormed infusion pump will be needed to deliver chemotherapy through this second catheter.

LEFT HEPATIC OFF LEFT GASTRIC (FIGURE 5)

If there is a replaced left hepatic artery originating from the left gastric, it will be necessary to place a catheter into the ascending or descending branch of the left gastric artery to perfuse the left lobe via the left hepatic artery. Ligation of this branch has not resulted in good collateral perfusion to supply the left lobe of the liver (Fig. 5).

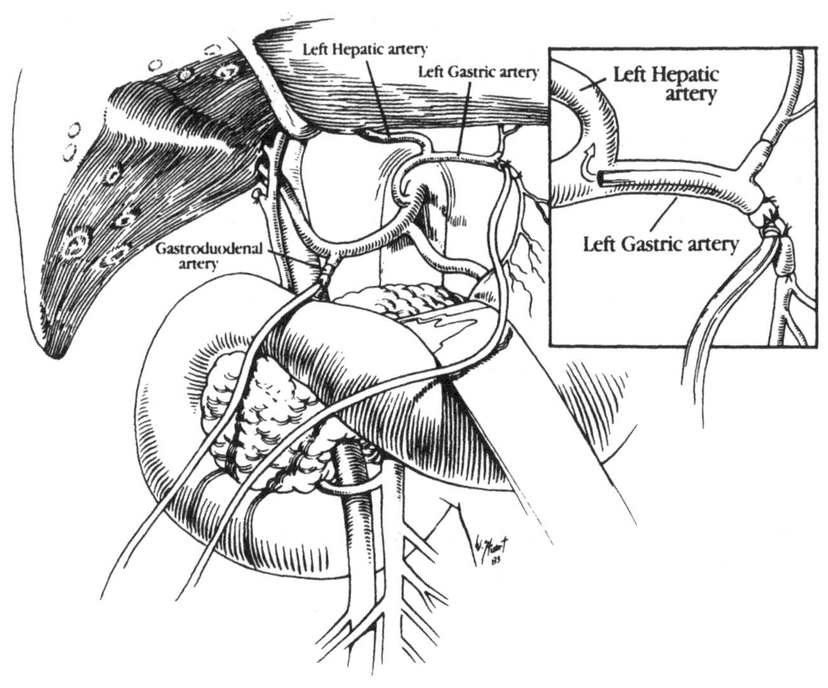

(FIGURE 5): LEFT HEPATIC OFF LEFT GASTRIC. Catheters placed into gastroduodenal artery and branch of left gastric.

TRIFURCATION OF COMMON HEPATIC ARTERY (FIGURE 6)

If the gastroduodenal artery origin is too close to the bifurcation of the proper hepatic artery, there will be insufficient mixing of drug perfusing both the right and left hepatic lobes. In this situation, the gastroduodenal artery should be ligated and the catheter placed via the proximal splenic artery into the common hepatic artery.

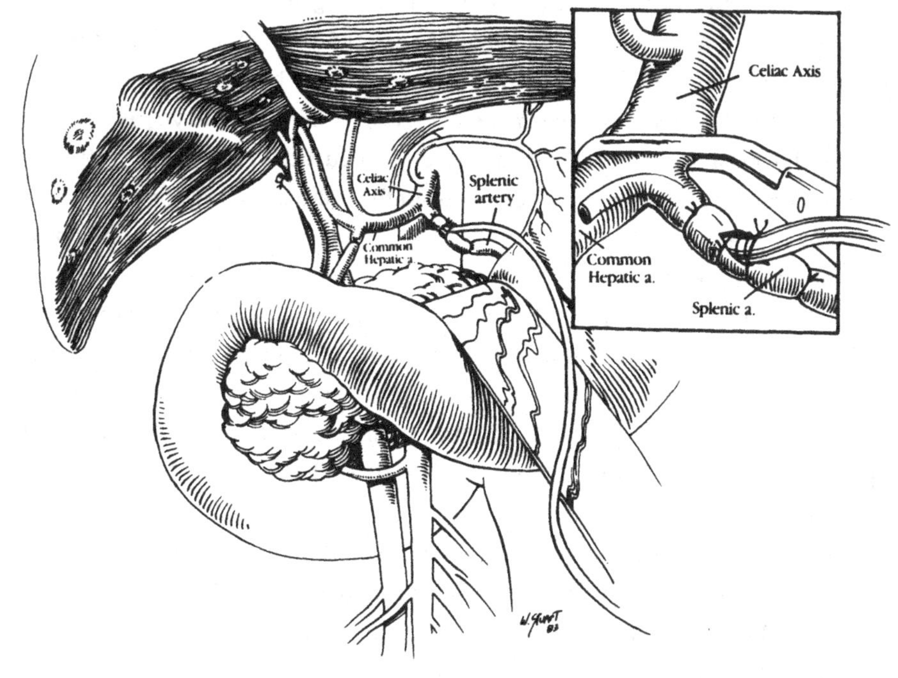

(FIGURE 6): TRIFURCATION OF COMMON HEPATIC INTO RIGHT AND LEFT HEPATIC AND GASTRODUODENAL ARTERY. Catheter placed via splenic into common hepatic with ligation of gastroduodenal artery.

The entire common hepatic artery should be skeletonized down to the celiac axis. Small pancreatic branches, if encountered, should be individually ligated. The celiac axis is isolated, and the splenic artery is skeletonized for 3 to 4 cm. The splenic artery is ligated 3 to 4 cm. from the take-off on the celiac axis. A Pilling clamp or Reynolds-Satinsky clamp is placed across the celiac axis - common hepatic junction above the left gastric take-off (Figure 6). A McFadden clip is placed across the common hepatic artery to prevent back flow. An anterior arteriotomy is made using a #11 blade and enlarged using Pott scissors. In some instances, the arteriotomy needs to be extended down the splenic artery across into the common hepatic to place the catheter. The arteriotomy in the latter case will need to be repaired using #5-0 or #6-0 Prolene suture after the catheter is placed. If the pump catheter passes easily into the common hepatic artery through the arteriotomy, this extension will not be necessary. In the latter case, a 3 to 4 cm. length of catheter proximal to the bead will be necessary. The bead is placed just inside the arteriotomy and the catheter tip directed into the common hepatic artery. Using several #2-0 silk sutures encompassing the splenic artery proximal and distal to the catheter bead, the catheter is secured in place. Perfusion is checked using Technetium 99 macroaggregated albumin perfusion scan.

Postoperatively, Technetium 99 MAA scan is performed to confirm that the catheter is perfusing the entire liver. Serial 360 degree projections around the liver and upper abdomen are obtained. The camera is then placed over the lungs and the lower abdomen to ensure that other organs are not unduly exposed to the intra-arterial drug. Perfusion scans are performed every two to three months during treatment to document the adequacy of perfusion and to identify any flow shifts that result in change in response.

If the right and left hepatic originate from the celiac, or there is early take-off of the left hepatic with the gastroduodenal arising from the right (Fig. 2B), then the pump catheter must be placed via the left gastric or splenic artery into the proximal common hepatic. If there is reversal of flow into the proper hepatic artery via the gastroduodenal artery secondary to arcuate ligament obstruction or thrombosis of the common hepatic artery (Fig. 1B), then the catheter should be placed through an anterior arteriotomy into the proximal hepatic artery and the catheter tip placed past the gastroduodenal - common hepatic junction. Intraoperative Technetium perfusion scan should be performed. If the gastroduodenal artery is ligated in the latter situation, the blood supply to the liver will be interrupted.

PERCUTANEOUS PLACEMENT

If the patient has had previous manipulation to the porta hepatis and has received x-ray therapy to this area or is a poor surgical candidate, then percutaneous placement of a #4 polyethylene arteriogram catheter, which is then connected to the implantable pump or portal, can be performed. (12) In the X-ray Department and under local anesthesia, a #4 polyethylene arteriogram catheter is placed via the left brachial artery and passed into the common hepatic artery beyond the gastroduodenal artery take-off.

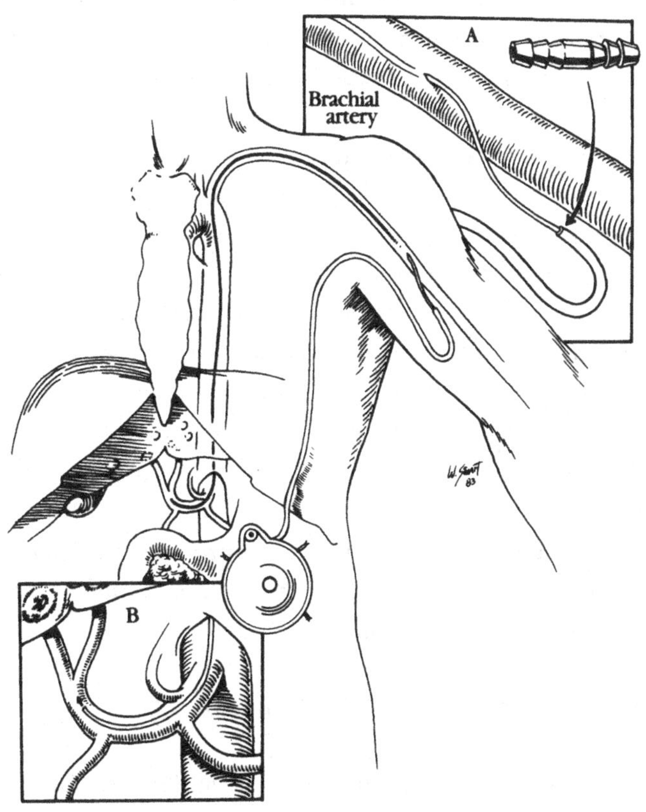

(FIGURE 7): TRANSBRACHIAL PLACEMENT OF HEPATIC ARTERY CATHETER WITH CONNECTION TO IMPLANTABLE PUMP.

In some cases, embolization of accessory or replaced arteries will be necessary. The catheter is connected to the external pumping device and the patient transferred to the Operating Room where connection to the Infusaid implantable pump or port is performed. (Figure 7). The pump is prepared in the usual manner and a pump pocket fashioned in the left upper quadrant below the left costal margin. If a portal is used, a pocket should be made in the lower sternal areas. A small skin incision is made at the lateral border of the pectoralis major muscle. The pump or portal is placed into the pocket and the catheter tunnelled to the left pectoral region. The catheter is passed from the pump or portal pocket through the subcutaneous tissues out the left pectoral incision. A 2.5 cm. transverse incision is made at the level of the catheter skin puncture site. The incision is carried down through the subcutaneous tissue to the fascia. A subcutaneous pocket is made beneath the distal portion of the incision. A connector is placed onto the end of the pump catheter and secured with #3-0 silk suture. The catheter is then tunnelled from the pectoral region to the catheter site. The polyethylene catheter is transected and the pump catheter and connector connected to the arteriogram catheter (See Insert, Fig. 7). The pump catheter is placed into the subcutaneous pocket of the upper arm so that it is doubled back on itself and then connected to the arteriogram catheter (Fig. 7). Using image intensification, the side port is flushed with Renografin and the flow into the hepatic artery ascertained. If the catheter is in an improper location or if a postoperative perfusion scan demonstrates flow into the G.I. tract or differential perfusion into the right or left lobe, the catheter should be repositioned while the patient is in the X-ray Department. If the X-ray suite is suitable, the entire procedure can be performed there under relatively sterile conditions. In both latter situations, the pump can be filled with chemotherapy at the onset.

POSTOPERATIVE FOLLOW-UP - INTRA-ARTERIAL

Postoperative follow-up includes intravenous antibiotics for 24 hours. A Technetium 99 MAA perfusion scan should be performed prior to discharge. Postoperative studies include CT scan of the liver and perfusion scans of the liver every two to three months. Liver function tests should be performed every two weeks. Significant neutropenia or thrombocytopenia have not been seen. FUDR at a dose of 0.2-0.3 mg/kg/day is infused every two weeks alternating with Heparin and water. Significant incidence of chemical hepatitis manifested by right upper quadrant pain, anorexia, nausea and elevation in liver function tests has been seen. If this occurs, the patient must be rested until the liver function tests improve. Chemotherapy is reinstituted at a reduced dose and slowly escalated. Oral steroids have been useful in ameliorating the symptoms of chemical hepatitis. Carafate, one gram every six hours by mouth, or Cimetadine have also been used during chemotherapy infusions. In a few instances where the Technetium 99 macroaggregated perfusion scan demonstrates significant shunting to the lungs, a few patients have developed chemical enteritis. If one suspects the latter entity (manifested by leukocytosis and severe diarrhea), the pump should be emptied immediately and replaced with Heparin and water. If the diarrhea persists, the patient should be made NPO and started on hyperalimentation. The latter may be required for six to eight weeks until the G.I. tract repairs itself. Steroids should also be used. Gastroscopy, including duodenoscopy and colonoscopy with biopsy, may be helpful in making the diagnosis. The Technetium 99 macroaggregated perfusion scan should be performed in all cases to make sure the catheter has not changed position.

Cholecystectomy is now routinely performed at the time of catheter and pump placement because of the high incidence of acalculus cholecystitis (40%). Ultrasound fails to demonstrate dilated biliary ducts or stones. Hyda scan is more reliable in making the diagnosis of acalculus cholecystitis. All patients presenting with this entity have had relief of symptoms when cholecystectomy was performed. After intra-arterial chemotherapy has been carried out for a long period of time, periportal fibrosis may develop, leading to common duct obstruction. This usually results in an increased bilirubin and alkaline phosphatase. Ultrasound has not been helpful in demonstrating this lesion since the liver is fibrotic and prevents ductal dilatation. A transhepatic cholangiogram is the best tool utilized in making the diagnosis. Transhepatic cholangiogram has demonstrated extrahepatic obstruction which, in over 50% of the cases, was secondary to periportal fibrosis rather than tumor. This entity is also seen in patients with percutaneously placed catheters. Decompression is best accomplished using transhepatic biliary drainage. Permanent internal biliary stents in most cases have lead to continuing sepsis and hepatic abscess. At the present time, decompressive external biliary tubes should be used since, if they become infected, they can be exchanged easily. Once these catheters are inserted, one is limited to the amount and duration of chemotherapy that can be administered intra-arterially.

VENOUS PLACEMENT

The best location for placement of a catheter for infusional therapy is the subclavian vein or internal jugular vein. If there is obstruction of the superior vena cava or subclavian vein secondary to tumor, the catheter can be placed through the saphenous vein into the inferior vena cava. In the latter situation the portal is located in the lower costal region.

The best and easiest method of placing the catheter into the superior vena cava is through the subclavian vein. This can be performed under local anesthesia. A #18 gauge needle is introduced into the subclavian vein through which a guide wire is directed into the superior vena cava under fluoroscopic control. A portal pocket is made in the lower sternal region. The catheter is tunnelled from the pocket out an incision made around the guide wire in the infraclavicular region. The catheter is trimmed so that the tip will lie in the superior vena cava. A peel-away catheter and obturator are then introduced over the guide wire, and when this reaches the superior vena cava, the obturator and guide wire are removed. The silastic catheter is introduced through the peel-away catheter into the superior vena cava. The introducer catheter is removed by peeling it apart, leaving the silastic catheter in place. The portal is secured in the pocket and the incisions closed. Infusions can be initiated at this time by leaving a Huber needle in place and connecting this to an infusion device.

AMBULATORY INFUSION

To carry out intra-arterial or intravenous infusional chemotherapy through a portal device, it will be necessary to use an external pumping device (13) to deliver the chemotherapy. The portal site is prepped with antiseptic scrub and solution. An angled (90°) 22 gauge Huber needle* is introduced through the skin into the portal system. The needle is flushed with heparin solution using a 5 or 10 cc. syringe. After proper position is ascertained, an extension tubing, preferably with a luer lock, is attached to the needle. This catheter is connected to the external pumping device catheter. A transparent adhesive dressing is placed over the site. The needle should be changed every five days. When the catheter and portal are not being used, it should be flushed with 3 cc. of heparin (1000 units/ml) once a week.

---

* Infusaid Corporation - Norwood, Mass.
Pharmacia Laboratories - Piscataway, N.J.

REFERENCES

1. Cady, B.: Hepatic arterial potency and complications after catheterization for infusion chemotherapy. Ann Surg (178): 156-161, 1973.
2. Clouse, M.E., Ahmed, R., Ryan, R.B., et al: Complications of long-term transbrachial hepatic arterial infusion chemotherapy. Am J Roentgenol (129): 799-803, 1977.
3. Dorr, R.T., Trinca, C.E., Griffith, R., et al: Limitations of a portable infusion pump in ambulatory patients receiving continuous infusions of anticancer drugs. Cancer Treatment Rep (63): 211, 213, 1979.
4. Grage, T.B., Vassiloupoulis, P.P., Shingleton, W.W., et al: Results of a prospective randomized study of hepatic artery infusion with 5-Fluorouracil versus intravenous 5-Fluorouracil in patients with hepatic metastases from colorectal cancer. Central Oncology Group Study, Surgery (86): 550-55, 1979.
5. Niederhuber, J.E., Ensminger, W., Gyves, J., et al: Regional chemotherapy of colorectal cancer metastatic to liver cancer. In press. Cancer.
6. Balch, C.M., Urist, M.M., Soong, S., et al: A prospective phase II clinical trial of continuous FUDR regional chemotherapy for colorectal metastases to the liver using a totally implantable pump. Am Surg (198): 567-573, 1983.
7. Barone, R.M., Byfield, J.E., Goldfarb, P.M., et al: Intra-arterial chemotherapy using an implantable infusion pump and liver irradiation for the treatment of hepatic metastases. Cancer (50): 850-862, 1982.
8. Blackshear, P.J., Rohde, T.D., Varco, R.L., et al: One year of continuous heparinization in the dog using a totally implanted infusion pump. SGO (141): 176-186, 1975.
9. Nebesar, R.A., Kornblith, P.L., Pollard, J.J., et al: In: Celiac and Superior Mesenteric Arteries. Anatomic Considerations. Little, Brown and Company, Boston, 1969, pp 9-34.
10. Bhargava, K.N., Rao, C.C.S., Aziz, M.H.A.: A study of hepatic arterial pattern in one hundred cadavers. Indian J Med Sci (34): 293-7, 1980.
11. Yang, P., Tuscan, M., Thrall, J.H., et al: Tc99m macroaggregated albumin perfusion scintiography for intraoperative hepatic artery chemotherapy catheter placement. J. Nuc Med (23): 1066-1069, 1982.
12. Cohen, A.M., Wood, W.C., Greenfield, G., et al: Transbrachial hepatic arterial chemotherapy using an implanted infusion pump. Dis Colon Rectum (23): 223-7, 1980.
13. Lokich, J. and Ensminger, W.: Ambulatory pump infusion devices for hepatic artery infusion. Seminars in Oncology (10): 183-190, 1983.

MANAGEMENT, COMPLICATIONS, AND EVALUATION OF INTRA-ARTERIAL INFUSIONS

WILLIAM D. ENSMINGER, PH.D., M.D.

INTRODUCTION

There are several elements which are unique to regional intra-arterial chemotherapy as compared to conventional systemic intravenous chemotherapy. One consideration is the need for a drug delivery system capable of infusing selected small arteries. Recent interest in intra-arterial chemotherapy has stemmed indirectly, in large part, from recent advances in drug delivery systems and monitoring, rather than from the discovery of new agents that are specifically more active when given intra-arterially[1]. Another unique aspect is that the toxicities of intra-arterial chemotherapy are generally different from the usual dose-limiting toxicities of systemic intravenous chemotherapy. A major nidus for toxicity is the intra-arterial drug delivery system itself. In addition, as one would anticipate from a regionally focused treatment, the major toxicities of intra-arterial treatment are regional in nature. This chapter will briefly review the major unique considerations with intra-arterial chemotherapy as commonly practiced.

DRUG DELIVERY SYSTEMS

There are essentially two major mechanisms for achieving intra-arterial access. These are angiographically or fluoroscopically positioned, relatively stiff, plastic catheters or surgically implantated silicone rubber (Silastic) catheters. In general, angiographically positioned catheters are useful for short term (minutes to hours) access since, in the long term, the frequency of arterial thrombosis rapidly rises with time[2]. Surgically placed silicone rubber catheters are much less thrombogenic and can be left in place for years, if required[3]. Table 1 lists the considerations that are important in the selection of the catheter system to be used in any individual patient or investigation. Angiographic placement of a catheter is much less traumatic to a patient, requires only a local anesthetic, and causes only short-term discomfort and minor cardiovascular stress from contrast dye injection. For a short-term infusion in a patient who could not readily withstand a major operation, but who has largely but not totally regionally confined tumor, angiographic placement is the method of choice. For a patient who has regionally confined tumor, who is in sufficiently good condition, and who is to receive a protracted treatment over months or years, the surgically placed catheter should be utilized. Catheters are usually connected to pumps to provide constant infusions. Angiographically positioned catheters are usually connected to external pumps, some of which are quite portable and convenient to use[4]. Surgically implanted catheters are frequently connected to an implanted pump. The Model 400 Infusaid pump (Infusaid, Norwood, MA) is the only FDA approved implantable pump commercially available, and literally thousands have been implanted for intra-arterial infusions. For purposes of discussion below, angiographic system will mean a system consisting of a percutaneous catheter positioned angiographically and attached to an external pump, a surgically implanted system will be one consisting of a silicone rubber catheter positioned into a vessel with an arterotomy, sutured in place, and then attached to an Infusaid Model 400 pump.

Table 1. Considerations in Selection of Angiographic Versus Surgically Implanted Drug Delivery Systems

1. Chronic versus short term
2. Skill of angiographer and surgeon
3. Experience/commitment of team
4. Region/organ infused
5. Stage/confinement of tumor
6. Condition of patient
7. Drugs
    a. Compatibility
    b. Stability
    c. Solubility

The complications and management considerations of the two types of drug delivery systems are noted on Table 2. The complication rate with either system is inversely proportional to the skill and commitment of the physicians involved. The use of Tc99m-macroaggregated albumin perfusion scans has become common for most regional intra-arterial infusions (except for brain) and allows definition of whether infusion to the entire region and all tumor in the region is being achieved[5].

Table 2. Complications and Management Considerations With Angiographic Versus Implanted Systems

	Complication	Frequency in System Angio	Surgical	Management Considerations
1.	Disruption of Infusion	Un-common	Uncommon	Pumps, lines, one-way valves, filters
2.	Inadequate Coverage with In-fusion	Common	Less	Catheter position and movement, un-identified vessels, thrombosis
3.	Thrombosis	Common	Uncommon	Catheter position, duration of in-fusion, blood flow reduction and dis-turbance, use of heparin and streptokinase to prevent and reverse, re-spectively
4.	Bleeding	Common	Uncommon	Catheter stability, one-way valve
5.	Infection	Infrequent	Less Frequent	Prophylactic anti-biotics, occlusive dressing

REGIONAL TOXICITIES

Achievement of much higher regional drug exposures generally leads to a higher rate of regional toxicities, with a variably lower rate of systemic toxicities. Table 3 lists the major regional toxicities described with effective intra-arterial drug treatments. The development of localized toxicities is, in fact, a verification of the higher regional drug exposure achieved by direct intra-arterial drug infusion. Management of the multiple complications of the many drug regimens used in the various body regions listed in Table 3 is beyond the scope of this presentation. Certain principles apply to all, however. First, most intra-arterial treatments probably are best treated as clinical investigation and should not be given, in general, by personnel who are unable to monitor the patient closely. Appropriate dose-schedule changes may decrease the incidence of toxicity. For example, with hepatic arterial infusions, decreasing the dose of fluorodeoxyuridine or giving a one-week instead of a two-week infusion can make it possible to prevent recurrence of hepatitis or gastritis and still effectively treat the patient. Attempts to selectively cannulate the tumor or to divert drug flow away from certain normal tissues are also useful.

Table 3. Toxicities as Related to Region/Organ Infused.

A. Brain
   1. Retinal damage/blindness in eye getting direct infusion
   2. Brain necrosis
   3. Ischemia due to vascular damage or emboli
   4. Dermatitis over forehead

B. Head and neck
   1. Mucositis
   2. Dermatitis
   3. Ulceration/abcess formation

C. Liver
   1. Hepatitis
   2. Gastritis
   3. Sclerosing cholangitis

D. Pelvic
   1. Cystitis
   2. Proctitis
   3. Mucositis/dermatitis
   4. Myelosuppression

E. Extremity
   1. Dermatitis/ulceration
   2. Myositis/neuritis
   3. Ischemia-claudication if vasculitis/ thrombosis

RESPONSE EVALUATION

Table 4 gives the usual measures of response evaluation and points out the problems with each. It must be noted that regionally toxic effects may be indistinguishable from progressive tumor. Nuclide and CT scans are indirect measures of tumor bulk. Direct visualization is preferable but not practical for most regionally confined tumors. Due to the great deal of extra effort, risk, and expense, one can conclude that only when cure is produced where none was generated with prior treatments, or only when survival is significantly increased as demonstrated by a randomized, controlled study, can one say that a regional therapy is efficacious in the strictest sense. It is usually true, however, that reductions in tumor volume demonstrated by a variety of methods are prerequisite for prolonged survival. Thus, improved response rates in refractory tumors determined by a variety of methods always generate considerable interest.

Table 4. Methods for Response Evaluation.

A. Nuclide scans--generally relate to vascular differences between tumor and normal surrounding tissue, low resolution.

B. CT scan--differences in tissue density and vascularity important, higher resolution, potentially overly sensitive.

C. Tumor markers--useful primarily in colorectal/GI cancer, depends on tumor differentiation, quantitative relevance in heterogenous tumors dubious.

D. Performance status--toxicity and tumor effects may be indistinguishable.

E. Organ function--toxicity and tumor effects may be indistinguishable.

F. Surgical--direct visualization/palpation not practical in most instances.

G. Survival--clean, but many variables generally uncontrolled or uncontrollable.

SUMMARY

The use of intra-arterial therapy is not nearly as easy as the use of systemic intravenous therapy. The unique complications of intra-arterial therapy can be minimized by selecting the right drug delivery system and by judicious use of appropriate chemotherapeutic agents. Intra-arterial therapy should not be used by physicians who are unwilling to provide the commitment necessary. Experience and dedication are essential ingredients. Only careful clinical investigation can underwrite the future in this area.

REFERENCES

1. Ensminger WD, Gyves JW: Regional cancer chemotherapy. Cancer Treat Rep (68):101-115, 1984.
2. Clouse ME, Ahmed R, Ryan RB, Oberfield RA, McCaffrey JA: Complications of long-term transbrachial hepatic arterial infusion chemotherapy. Am J Roentgenol (129):799-803, 1977.
3. Niederhuber JE, Ensminger WD, Gyves JW, Thrall J, Walker S, Cozzi E: Regional chemotherapy of colorectal cancer metastatic to the liver. Cancer (53):1336-1343, 1984.
4. Lokich J, Ensminger W: Ambulatory pump infusion devices for hepatic artery infusion. Sem Onc (10):183-190, 1983.
5. Kaplan WD, Ensminger WD, Come SE, Smith EH, D'Orsi CJ, Levin DC, Takvorian RW, Steele GD, Jr: Radionuclide angiography to predict patient response to hepatic artery chemotherapy. Cancer Treat Rep (64):1217-1222, 1980.

PHARMACOKINETIC RATIONALE FOR INTRACAVITARY THERAPY

JERRY M. COLLINS

1. INTRODUCTION

The field of intracavitary therapy has progressed so rapidly over the last few years that this conference has the luxury of separate coverage for theory and experimental results. Other presentations will focus on the clinical and pharmacokinetic results of intracavitary trials, so I'll focus mainly on the background and theory. In particular, I have been asked to cover those pharmacokinetic factors which led to the pursuit of intracavitary therapy.

When we use the term "intracavitary" at this conference, the peritoneal and pleural spaces are the first to come to mind. The next areas might be the brain, pericardium, and urinary bladder. Although the brain is not the first area that many would list for intracavitary therapy, it should be recognized that the most widely accepted indication for intracavitary treatment is meningeal disease, especially for acute lymphoblastic leukemia.

The majority of this presentation will focus upon intraperitoneal therapy, but these concepts can be readily generalized to the pleural space and other areas of the body.

2. INTRAPERITONEAL THERAPY: CONCEPTUAL BASIS

Our efforts at NCI were by no means the first attempts at intraperitoneal therapy, but we were the first group to recognize the necessity of administering drugs in a LARGE volume so that ALL potential intraabdominal sites of disease were exposed. Subsequent to our revival of clinical interest in intraperitoneal therapy, other groups have made substantial contributions and their work is covered in other presentations at this conference.

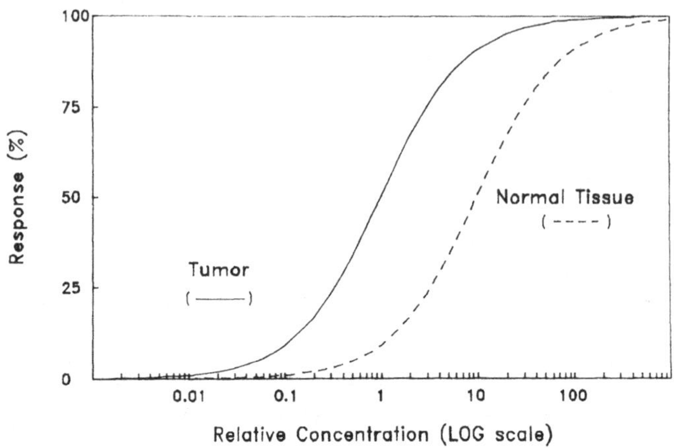

FIGURE 1. Response vs. concentration relationship for a typical drug. Solid line is for tumor, dashed line is for normal host tissue.

The first disease which we at NCI decided to approach was ovarian carcinoma. Dr. Vincent DeVita recognized that this disease was confined to the abdominal space for most of its natural history, but the limiting toxicity for chemotherapy was in organs outside the desired treatment area, such as bone marrow or gastrointestinal mucosa. Dr. DeVita proposed intraperitoneal delivery of anticancer drugs as a strategy to improve the therapeutic index. Subsequently, our group and others have recognized that the same characteristics apply to some forms of colon cancer and mesothelioma.

The goal of intracavitary therapy is to achieve higher concentrations at the target site than would be possible with the use of systemic drug delivery. As shown in Figure 1, it is expected that higher drug concentrations will result in increased antitumor effect, so long as the maximum effect has not yet been reached. Toxicity to normal tissues will also increase as the concentration increases, which limits the maximum concentration that can be achieved with systemic therapy. Conceptually, the intracavitary approach is an attempt to increase the separation between the two curves in Figure 1.

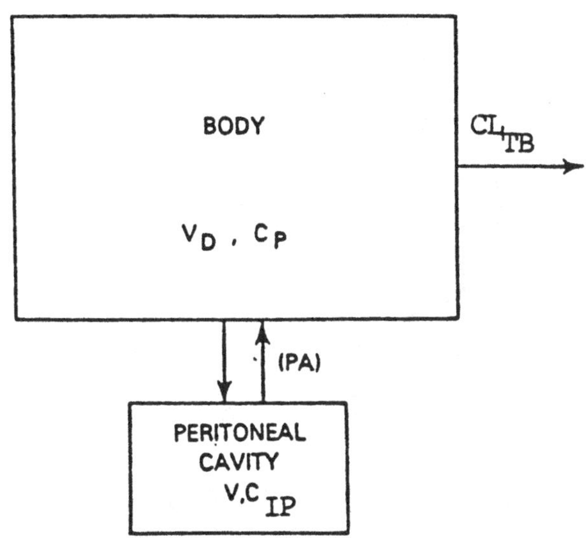

FIGURE 2. Two-compartment model for intraperitoneal drug delivery.

3. PHARMACOKINETIC MODELING OF INTRAPERITONEAL THERAPY

In addition to the focus upon large fluid volumes, another unique feature of our intraperitoneal effort at NCI was the complete pharmacokinetic description of intraperitoneal therapy. In fact, the galley proofs of the initial modeling paper by Dedrick et al. (1) were prepared BEFORE the first patient was treated. This paper has just been recognized as one of the most cited works in Cancer Treatment Reports (2).

Figure 2 is a diagram of the basic 2-compartment model (1) which is used for the analysis of intraperitoneal drug delivery. A peritoneal compartment is created by the instillation of 2 liters of dialysis fluid. The drug can be pre-mixed in the dialysis fluid or can be given as a constant infusion into the peritoneum. We can use this model (Figure 2) to predict R_d, the ratio of peritoneal fluid and plasma concentrations for intraperitoneal drug delivery:

Steady-State Infusion	Intermittent (Bolus)
$R_d = \frac{C_{IP}}{C_p} = 1 + \frac{CL_{TB}}{PA}$	$R_d = \frac{AUC_{IP}}{AUC_p} = 1 + \frac{CL_{TB}}{PA}$

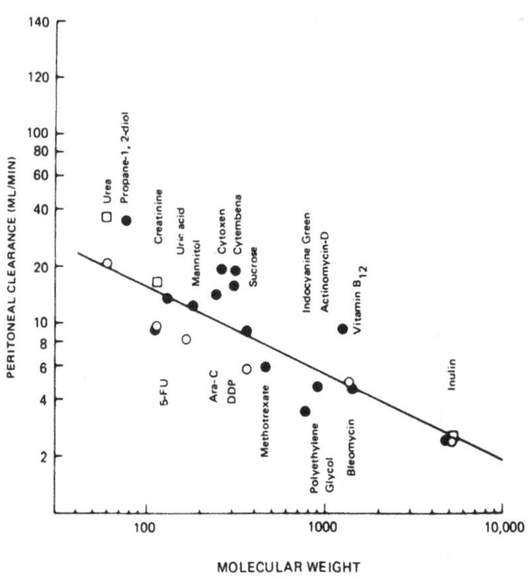

FIGURE 3. Log-log plot of peritoneal clearance vs. molecular weight. Open symbols, human data; solid circles, rat data scaled according to surface area. From reference (3).

The form of these equations is very similar to the analogous equations for intraarterial and intrathecal drug delivery (4). Only 2 parameters are needed for each drug: CL_{TB} and PA. CL_{TB} is the total body clearance, which can be obtained from published reports for intravenous doses. PA is the peritoneal clearance or permeability-area product, which is a new quantity. Unlike blood flow in the analogous equation for intraarterial delivery, this quantity could not be found in a textbook, at least at the time in which the first intraperitoneal trials were conducted.

For the initial human trials, PA was estimated from a log-log plot of PA vs. molecular weight. PA values were known for a few compounds (physiological markers) from studies of peritoneal dialysis in patients with kidney disease. As shown in Figure 3, these human experimental values were supplemented by the data from a series of experiments in which intraperitoneal anticancer drugs were given to rats (5). The rat values were adjusted to human dimensions by assuming that peritoneal surface area followed the same scaling laws as external body surface area. As we have acquired actual human data for anticancer drugs, we have verified

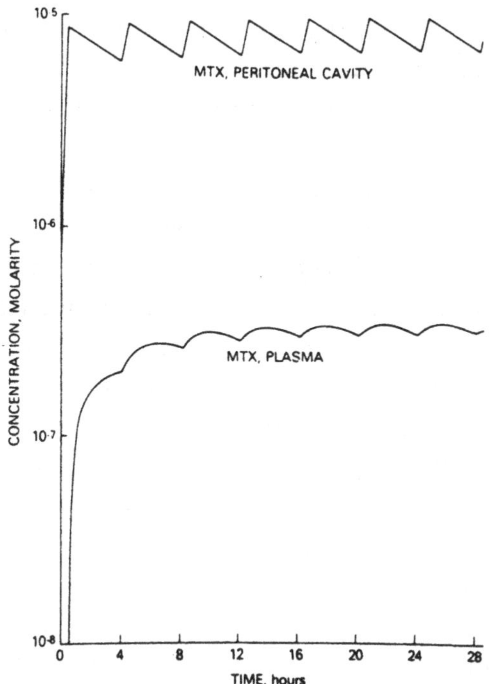

FIGURE 4. Predicted pharmacokinetic behavior for MTX in plasma and peritoneal fluid following intraperitoneal delivery (1). Initial peritoneal fluid concentration was 9 μM.

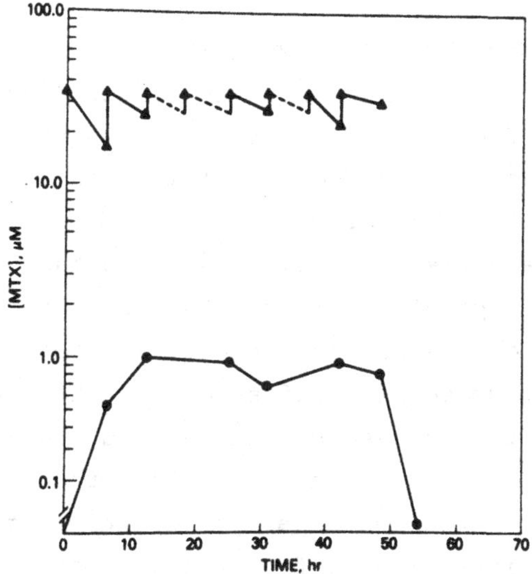

FIGURE 5. Measured concentrations of MTX during intraperitoneal therapy (6). Initial peritoneal fluid concentration was 35 μM.

the suitability of this estimation process. It should be stressed that this correlation applies only to hydrophillic substances. Lipophillic compounds would be cleared (absorbed) at a much faster rate.

The initial theoretical paper (1) had predicted the pharmacokinetics of intraperitoneal methotrexate (MTX, Figure 4), and this was the first drug tested clinically. We knew in advance that the intraperitoneal route would produce substantially higher peritoneal fluid concentrations of MTX than the intravenous route, though not as high as some other drugs. An additional consideration in the selection of MTX was the element of safety, especially the availability of leucovorin rescue and the knowledge that MTX penetrated ascitic effusions when given systemically. Thus, peritoneal surfaces were exposed to MTX during systemic therapy without limiting toxicity.

The intraperitoneal MTX clinical results (6) are shown in Figure 5. Although there are differences in the MTX dose and some parameter values between the simulations in Figure 4 and the data in Figure 5, the general level of agreement, primarily the peritoneal fluid:plasma concentration difference, is excellent. Other groups at this conference will cover additional drugs.

4. DIFFUSION DISTANCE/PENETRATION DEPTH

Conceptually, we realize that the closer a tumor cell is to the peritoneal fluid, the higher its exposure. But what are the quantitative dimensions: how small is "minimal" disease and how large is "bulky" disease?

We can approach these quantitative aspects with mathematical modeling, but the type of model is rather different from the compartmental approaches used to predict peritoneal fluid concentrations. As drug molecules diffuse out of the peritoneal cavity and into tissues, they cross capillaries and are washed away by blood. Thus, blood flow acts as a "sink" for the drug. Drug concentration in the tissues adjacent to the peritoneal cavity depends upon the <u>distance</u> away from the peritoneal cavity as well as time. This type of model is shown in Figure 6.

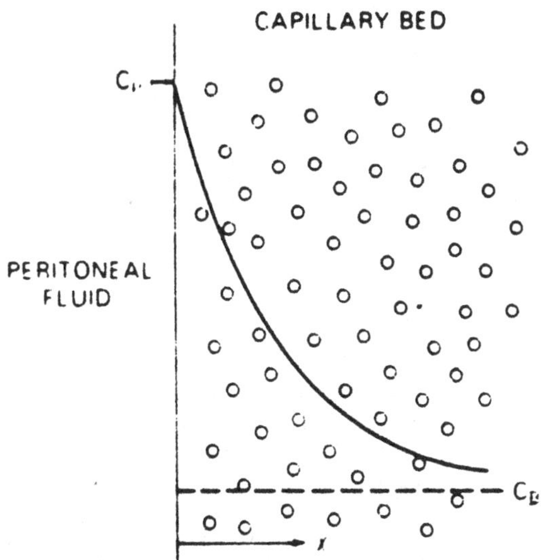

FIGURE 6. Distributed model for peritoneal drug delivery (7). Theoretical description of tissue concentration profile.

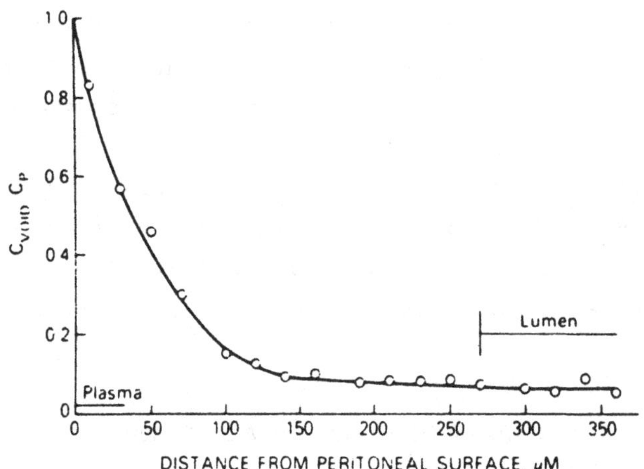

FIGURE 7. Concentration profile in jejunal tissue in the rat (7). Comparison between experimental data (o) and model simulations (solid line) for polyethylene glycol-900.

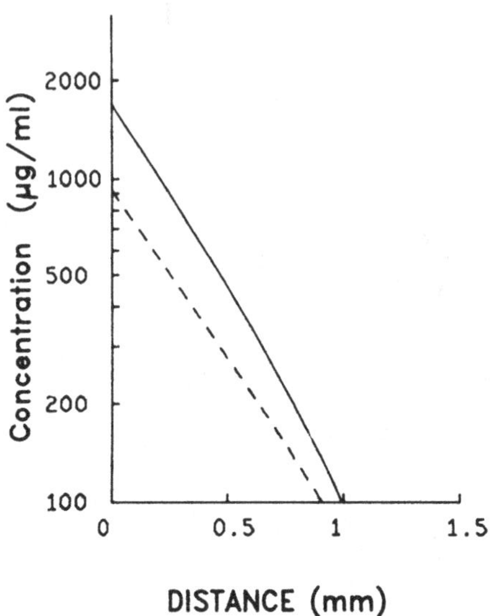

FIGURE 8. Model simulation of the development of a distance profile. Solid line is profile at 30 minutes; dashed line is profile at 3 hours. From reference (8).

Although this theoretical approach is not easy, it should be recognized that experimental approaches are also quite difficult. The only set of data which I am aware of were generated by Michael Flessner for his Ph.D. thesis. A sample of his data is shown in Figure 7. In addition to the qualitative agreement with the general behavior suggested by Figure 6, Flessner was also able to quantitatively determine model parameters, as shown by the agreement between the data and simulations.

The concentration in peritoneal tissues varies with both position and time. Figure 8 is a simulation presented as part of a study of intraperitoneal misonidazole (8). The simulation suggests that it takes about 30 minutes to fully develop the distance profile.

5. USE OF INTRAPERITONEAL THERAPY AS AN ALTERNATIVE TO HEPATIC ARTERY CANNULATION

The intraperitoneal route has also been used to deliver drugs to tumor cells in the liver (9). When these studies were first proposed in 1977, the technical barriers to hepatic artery infusion were far more imposing than they are in 1984. Since it had always been thought that intraperitoneal drug is absorbed via the hepatic portal vein, the intraperitoneal approach was viewed as a more technically feasible alternative to hepatic arterial (or portal vein) infusions. It is important to note that this approach can treat both local peritoneal disease as well as hepatic disease. Of course, for large hepatic metastases, many would say that intraportal approaches are inappropriate, since the tumor's circulation is derived from the hepatic artery. In any event, the basic assumption of portal drainage and quantification of drug levels which could be achieved in the hepatic circulation had never been documented. Therefore, we undertook a clinical pharmacokinetic study with intraperitoneal 5-FU in which sampling catheters were placed in the peritoneal fluid, portal vein, hepatic vein, peripheral artery, and peripheral vein.

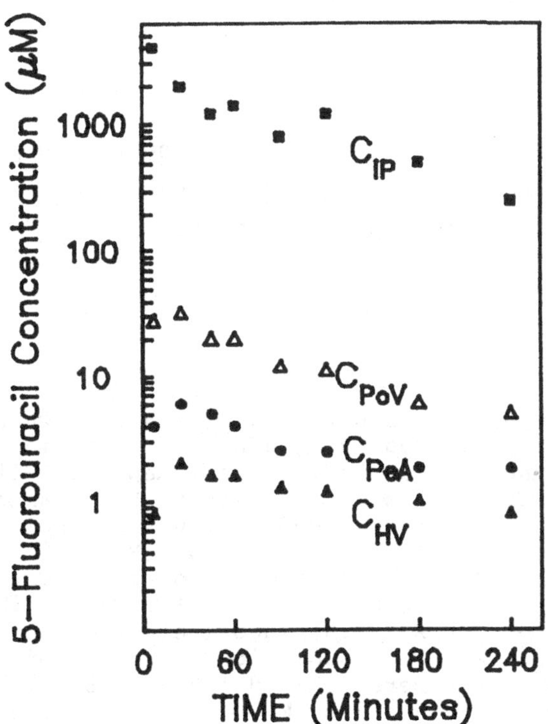

FIGURE 9. Concentrations of 5-FU in the peritoneal fluid (C_{IP}), portal vein (C_{PoV}), hepatic vein (C_{HV}), and peripheral artery (C_{PeA}). Data from reference (9).

As illustrated in Figure 9, portal vein concentrations of 5-FU averaged 4 times as high as peripheral arterial 5-FU concentrations. Thus, the intraperitoneal route provides an effective way to increase hepatic 5-FU delivery, at least for tumors nourished by the portal vein.

6. INTRACAVITARY CONCEPTS: APPLICATION TO INTRATHECAL THERAPY

Intrathecal therapy for meningeal leukemia is the most widely accepted indication for intracavitary therapy. Dedrick and coworkers (10) described intrathecal MTX delivery with a compartmental model which was very similar to the one shown in Figure 2 for intraperitoneal delivery. Although the intrathecal route has had demonstrable success for treating meningeal disease, one must keep in mind that parenchymal brain tumors can't be successfully treated with this approach. The concept of penetration depth (distributed model) has been ably presented for intraventricular therapy by Blasberg and colleagues (11).

7. ACKNOWLEDGEMENTS

The work described herein would not have been possible without the combined efforts of many investigators at NIH, especially Robert Dedrick and Charles Myers.

REFERENCES

1. Dedrick RL, Myers CE, Bungay PM, DeVita VT: Pharmacokinetic rationale for peritoneal drug administration in the treatment of ovarian cancer. Cancer Treatment Rep. 62:1-11, 1978.
2. Sloane EM, Baum JG, Hubbard SM, Wittes RE: Cancer Treatment Reports 1959-1983: Background review and tabular compilation of most-cited articles. Cancer Treat. Rep. 68:329-337, 1984.
3. Myers CE, Collins JM: Pharmacology of intraperitoneal chemotherapy. Cancer Investigation 1:395-407, 1983.
4. Collins JM, Dedrick RL: Pharmacokinetics of Anticancer Drugs. In: Chabner BA (ed) Pharmacologic Principles of Cancer Treatment, W.B. Saunders, Philadelphia, 1982, pp 77-99.
5. Jones RB, Myers CE, Guarino AM, Dedrick RL, Hubbard SM, DeVita VT: High-volume intraperitoneal chemotherapy ("belly bath") for ovarian cancer. Cancer Chemother. Pharmacol 1:161-166, 1978.

6. Jones RB, Collins JM, Myers CE, Brooks AE, Hubbard SM, Balow JE, Brennan MF, Dedrick RL, DeVita VT: High-volume intraperitoneal chemotherapy with methotrexate in patients with cancer. Cancer Res. 41:55-59, 1981.
7. Dedrick RL, Flessner MF, Collins JM, Schultz JS: Is the peritoneum a membrane? ASAIO J. 5:1-8, 1982.
8. Gianni L, Jenkins JF, Greene RF, Lichter AS, Myers CE, Collins JM: Pharmacokinetics of the hypoxic radiosensitizers misonidazole and desmethylmisonidazole after intraperitoneal administration in humans. Cancer Res. 43:913-916, 1983.
9. Speyer JL, Sugarbaker PH, Collins JM, Dedrick RL, Klecker RW, Myers CE: Portal levels and hepatic clearance of 5-fluorouracil after intraperitoneal administration in humans. Cancer Res. 41:1916-1922, 1981.
10. Dedrick RL, Zaharko DS, Bender RA, Bleyer WA, Lutz RJ: Pharmacokinetic considerations on resistance to anticancer drugs. Cancer Chemother. Rep. 59:795-804, 1975.
11. Blasberg R, Patlak CS, Fenstermacher JD: Intrathecal chemotherapy: Brain tissue profiles after ventriculocisternal perfusion. J. Pharmacol. Exp. Ther. 195:73-83, 1975.

SURGICAL PRINCIPLES OF INTRAPERITONEAL ACCESS AND THERAPY

WILLIAM E. LUCAS, M.D.

Paralleling the development of an effective system for treating intraperitoneal cancer with markedly augmented local concentrations of chemotherapeutic agents has been an evolving search for safe and effective techniques for maintaining chronic access to the peritoneal cavity.

Before describing these efforts in detail it is pertinent to review a rational overall approach to the treatment of advanced ovarian cancer. Aggressive primary surgery with the object of accurately defining the extent of disease and of reducing residual disease to the smallest aggregates possible, followed by systemic polychemotherapy, has resulted in significant improvements in survival time for patients with advanced (Stages III and IV) ovarian cancer during the last decade.[1] The dilemma has been how to best manage those patients found to have residual disease at the time of surgical re-exploration, i.e., those patients who have failed to achieve complete remission following first and/or second line systemic chemotherapy. Among the alternatives currently available are the use of different systemic drug therapy protocols, whole abdominal irradiation, and intraperitoneal chemotherapy.

Phase II studies to determine the efficacy of the intraperitoneal route have been under way at the University of California, San Diego, since 1980. Initially peritoneal access was achieved using standard chronic two cuff Tenckhoff catheters. Because of poor patient acceptability, high maintenance requirements, and risk of infection with the standard Tenckhoff system, since September 1982 a totally implantable system has been used. It is the purpose of this report to describe our experience with this system.

MATERIALS

Port-A-Cath (PAC) peritoneal portals (Part number 550-570) and 19 gauge Huber-point needles (Part number 550-744) were purchased from Pharmacia Nu Tech (Piscataway, New Jersey 08854). Catheters (Part number 008-173-000) were purchased from Coloe Laboratories, Inc., (Lakewood, Colorado 80215).

The PAC is a totally implantable system which permits repeated access to the peritoneal cavity. The system consists of three components: a stainless steel portal, a catheter, and a stainless steel slip lock for securing the catheter to the portal (Figure 1).

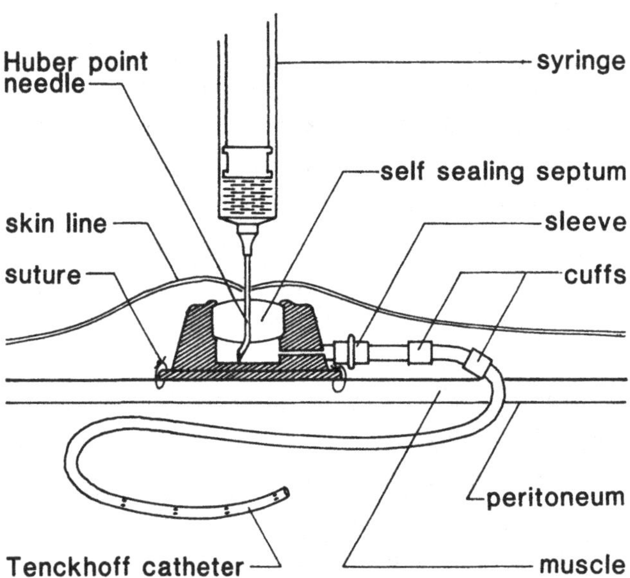

INFUSION CYCLE

The portal has a self-sealing implantable grade silicone septum positioned in the top. Entry into the portal is gained by the percutaneous placement of a Huber-point needle through the portal septum. The deflected point of the Huber needle prevents coring and hence preserves septal integrity.

We have found that the system which has worked best for us is to attach a chronic Tenckhoff catheter, using only the portion distal to the proximal Teflon cuff to the Port-A-Cath. The proximal end of the catheter is threaded through the steel slip lock, which then secures the catheter to the Port-A-Cath nozzle.

PATIENT SELECTION AND TECHNIQUE OF PLACEMENT

All of our patients who have been candidates for intraperitoneal chemotherapy have had two or more previous operations, and many have had gross residual disease and/or ascites. We prefer to place the PAC over the lower rib cage in the midclavicular line, which places the site of entry into the peritoneal cavity on the left or right side of the abdomen at, or just above, the level of the umbilicus. However, in the face of multiple previous operations and a history of intraperitoneal disease, finding a safe "window" into the peritoneal cavity is best done with the aid of ultrasonic screening. Obviously, the location of a safe site will determine the location of the PAC. It is desirable to have the firm support of the ribs behind the PAC to facilitate insertion of the Huber needle, and in actual practice it has almost always been possible to site the PAC over the lower rib cage.

The procedure can be done under local or general anesthesia. Our usual choice has been general anesthesia since it eliminates patient discomfort and allows more rapid catheter placement. Also, if easy entry into the peritoneal cavity is not achieved after attempts at two or more sites, laparotomy can be considered as an option in order to define the extent of adhesions and make a decision as to whether good catheter placement is possible in the first place. Inadvertent enterotomy is a potential complication of attempted entry into the peritoneal cavity because of adhesions due to previous surgery and/or the underlying disease. Although careful preoperative evaluation to select the best site for catheter placement, including sonographic or CT scanning and careful intraoperative technique should minimize the risk of damage to adherent bowel, the surgeon should be prepared to deal with this complication, and all patients should be prepared for possible laparotomy.

Ideally the intraperitoneal catheter should be placed at the time of re-exploration where obvious residual disease is found. However, for patients with recurrent disease after negative findings at previous re-exploration or patients referred for catheter placement, it is necessary to decide whether a third or fourth exploration is indicated to define the extent of disease and attempt further cytoreductive surgery. Careful review of the patient's history and appropriate non-invasive diagnostic studies will aid in making an appropriate decision. Since in this pilot study many of our patients have had several previous operations and often have had ascites and known widespread intraperitoneal disease, full-scale laparotomy has not often been considered appropriate However, "open" laparoscopy, using the Hassan cannula inserted via the peritoneal opening through which the intraperitoneal catheter is to be placed is an option that we have utilized. This affords a relatively simple and safe method for evaluating peritoneal and serosal surfaces for tumor implants and may make it possible to gauge the extent of pre-existing adhesions.

The actual technique of PAC and catheter placement involves first marking on the skin of either upper abdominal quadrant the sites for entry into the peritoneal cavity and for the PAC. The lower incision is made first, the anterior muscle fascia opened transversely, the muscles retracted, and the peritoneum opened. A chromic catgut pursestring suture is placed around the peritoneal opening, and the ends left long with needle still attached. The upper incision is carried down to deep fascia and a subcutaneous pocket made for the PAC. A long curved clamp is passed upward from the lower incision to make a subcutaneous tunnel for the catheter, which is brought down through the tunnel and inserted into the peritoneal cavity. The pursestring suture is tied just below the Teflon cuff and the cuff is further secured with the chromic suture. The muscle fascia is closed with a continuous polyglycolic suture, and the PAC is sutured to the deep fascia with similar sutures. The skin incisions are closed with subcuticular sutures. The PAC is filled with either heparinized saline or 20 ml of 32% Dextran-70 at the conclusion of the procedure.

CLINICAL EXPERIENCE

Between 9/2/82 and 12/15/83, sixty-one intraperitoneal PAC units have been placed and a total of 200 courses of chemotherapy delivered. In two patients referred for catheter placement, it was impossible to gain suitable access to the peritoneal cavity, and in an additional two referred patients no attempt to place a catheter was made because of the advanced stage of disease and poor performance status. In three cases early in our experience, it was necessary to replace two PACs and revise the position of a third because of improper placement or malfunction.

There have been no wound infections involving the subcutaneous tunnel and PAC implantation site. At some point in their course of intraperitoneal chemotherapy, five patients have developed bacterial peritonitis (4 due to staphylococcus epidermidis and 1 due to staphylococcus aureus). In three of these cases failure to respond to systemic and intraperitoneal antibiotic therapy has necessitated PAC removal. Two catheters have been removed at the time of laparotomies done because of intestinal obstruction, and one was removed at the patient's request.

In general, patient acceptance of the implanted PAC systems has been excellent. There has been virtually no limitation of activity attributable to the PAC.

One other complication of note was an instance of severe anaphylaxis three minutes after 20 ml of Dextran-70 had been injected into the PAC. Fortunately the patient had an endotracheal tube in place and recovered after appropriate resuscitation. At the present time, methods other than Dextran to prevent adhesions are being explored.

As noted above, two patients in this series required reoperation for intestinal obstruction due to marked adhesive disease after 4 and 3 courses of intraperitoneal chemotherapy, respectively. Since both patients had been subjected to laparotomy at the time of catheter placement (in one case a "second look" and in one a "third look") with only minimal to moderate adhesive disease present, it is assumed that the adhesions were at least in part due to a chemical peritonitis secondary to the drug therapy. Clinically, in both cases, a fibrous pseudomembrane encased multiple loops of small intestine, requiring a technically difficult dissection.

A more insidious problem related to the catheters is eventual inability to drain the peritoneal cavity via the PAC. To date, 13 out of 61 catheters have become one-way valves. This one-way valve effect is probably due to formation of a fibrous sheath and was the reason for using Dextran to flush the system after each injection of chemotherapy. However, it would appear from life-table analysis that approximately half of all the catheters eventually lose two-way function, and that the use of Dextran has not been effective.

The problem of adhesion formation, in terms of catheter function, in terms of preventing good distribution of drugs within the peritoneal cavity, and as a potential cause of major morbidity due to intestinal obstruction, remains unresolved. It would appear that Dextran is not very effective in preventing adhesions in the context of this system of intraperitoneal therapy. Recent research suggests that nonsteroidal anti-inflammatory drugs such as Ibuprofen may be of some value in preventing postsurgical adhesions.[2] The theory on which this therapy is proposed is that since arachidonic acid metabolites mediate the acute fibroproliferative inflammatory response following surgical trauma, high doses of an anti-arachidonic acid should suppress this response. It is to be hoped that appropriate clinical trials fulfill this promise.

COMMENT

Although the system described above for delivering intraperitoneal drugs has been relatively effective and trouble free, major improvement is needed to prevent the problems associated with adhesions around the catheter and elsewhere within the abdomen. The use of nonsteroidal anti-inflammatory drugs to lessen this problem will be explored. We believe that the problem of peritonitis, although potentially serious, can be held to a minimum by careful adherence to correct antiseptic technique. Several other catheters are available which could be used with the totally implantable PAC system. Two that appear promising and which should be compared to the Tenckhoff catheter are the Lifecath (Physio-Control Corporation, 11811 Willows Road, Redmond, Washington) and the Toronto Western Hospital catheter (OZ-TWH-99 DBC, Accurate Surgical Instruments Co., 588 Richmond Street West, Toronto, Ontario M5V 1Y9, Canada).

Since this has been a pilot study, the results of which will be discussed as a subsequent presentation in this symposium, patient selection has largely been based on overall suitability for surgery. As noted above, the only patients where no attempt has been made to place a catheter have had advanced disease and intestinal obstruction considered to be inoperable. Of those patients selected for attempted catheter placement using the totally implantable system, in only 2 out of 63 was it impossible to gain access to the peritoneal cavity.

In line with repeatedly documented results of treatment of advanced ovarian cancer with systemic chemotherapy, it is very likely that the best longterm results will be obtained where minimal residual disease is present when intraperitoneal chemotherapy is instituted.

REFERENCES

1. Berek JS, Hacker N, Lagasse LD: Recent progress in the treatment of epithelial ovarian malignancy. West J Med (137): 273-277, 1982.

2. Nishimura K, Nakamura RM, DiZerago GS: Ibuprofen inhibition of postsurgical adhesion formation: A time and dose response biochemical evaluation in rabbits. J Surg Res. To be published 1984

MEDICAL PRINCIPLES OF INTRAPERITONEAL AND INTRAPLEURAL CHEMOTHERAPY

MAURIE MARKMAN, M.D.

While modeling studies have suggested a major pharmacokinetic advantage for peritoneal cavity drug exposure to certain chemotherapeutic agents when administered by the intraperitoneal route (1), there are both theoretical and practical issues which must be addressed prior to the acceptance of this approach to the management of malignant disease principally confined to the peritoneal or pleural cavities. The importance of establishing a safe and simple method of accessing the abdominal cavity has been discussed in another paper in this symposium. Other questions to be addressed include:

1. Is there adequate drug distribution when drugs are administered intraperitoneally or intrapleurally? How can one assure as much exposure as possible?
2. Although direct tumor-drug interactions might be greater with intracavitary drug administration, is one compromising treatment efficacy by decreasing tumor exposure to drugs by capillary flow?
3. How can one prevent and treat the potential, unique complications of therapy, including chemical and bacterial peritonitis?
4. What are the optimal drugs, dosages, rates of drug administration and scheduling programs for the different tumors which might be approached by the intracavitary route?

As the surface area of the peritoneal cavity is significantly greater than the pleural cavity, the problem of adequate drug distribution is potentially more serious during intraperitoneal therapy. However, certain tumors which might involve the pleural cavity can elicit an intense fibrous reaction, which could make it difficult for instilled drug to reach all pleural-based tumor. In addition, patients previously treated with multiple thoracentesis to drain effusions or with chest tube drainage (with or without attempts at sclerosis) will likely have loculated pockets of fluid-containing tumor, making adequate drug distribution a difficult problem.

During intraperitoneal chemotherapy, the importance of the issue of drug distribution becomes central to the efficacy of this treatment approach. For example, ovarian carcinoma, one of the most common neoplasms to involve the abdominal cavity and remain localized to this region during most of its natural history, commonly seeds the whole of the peritoneal cavity as well as the rich lymphatic network on the undersurfaces of the diaphragms (2). Several studies have now demonstrated that drugs administered in small volumes (3-500 ml) <u>will not</u> be adequately distributed throughout all parts of the peritoneal cavity, in spite of the earlier assumption that the cavity is potentially free flowing. However, when <u>large volumes</u> are used to distend the abdominal cavity, excellent drug distribution can be achieved (3-5). For example, Rosenshein, et al., studying the distribution of ^{99}Tc labelled serum albumin following instillation into the peritoneal cavity of monkeys in volumes equivalent to 0.2% (10 ml) or 5% (250 ml) of their body weight, demonstrated that radioactivity was limited to only a portion of the cavity when the smaller volume was administered. In addition, neither vigorous massaging of the abdomen nor head-up or head-down tilting of the animal improved the distribution. When the larger volume was instilled, however, there was uniformly good distribution of the radioactivity throughout the abdomen. The same maneuvers of head-up and head-down tilting resulted in a shift of the whole distribution of the administered fluid (3).

Thus, the concept of administration of chemotherapeutic agents in large volumes has become a cornerstone for the successful application of the basic principles of intracavitary therapy. An added benefit of administering drugs in large rather than small volumes would be the prevention of the development of extremely high concentration pockets of drugs capable of producing focal necrosis (particularly of bowel or lung) or other serious toxicities.

In ovarian carcinoma or other malignancies where surgery has preceded intracavitary drug administration, the risk of adhesion formation and the establishment of loculated regions limiting the free flow of fluid are major concerns. In addition, tumors can themselves elicit an intense inflammatory reaction with significant fibrous tissue reaction and the development of adhesions. During a phase I trial of the intraperitoneal administration of cisplatin conducted at the UCSD Cancer Center, we investigated the distribution of ^{99}Tc-sulfur colloid instilled in two liters of saline in patients prior to drug administration. In seven of ten patients with advanced ovarian carcinoma who had undergone at least one laparotomy prior to entering this trial, the ^{99}Tc-sulfur colloid was distributed into all four quadrants when scanned shortly after instillation (6).

Similarly, Dunnick and his collaborators at the National Cancer Institute have examined the distribution of intraperitoneal Hypaque administered in large volumes to nine patients with ovarian carcinoma and one patient with peritoneal melanoma (7). In eight of the ten patients, the distribution was complete and unimpaired when patients were examined by computerized axial tomography. In addition, we have also demonstrated that even in some patients who demonstrate poor distribution when scanned shortly after fluid administration, if they are scanned several hours later, one notes the gradual appearance of contrast material into the areas where none had been previously observed. Finally, in several patients who intially did not demonstrate adequate distribution _prior to_ the initiation of therapy, when re-scanned following response to treatment, they have demonstrated improved fluid distribution. This would suggest that in certain patients the impaired distribution is at least partially due to the presence of tumor and that effective chemotherapy can allow treatment courses to reach previously inaccessible tumor.

Another concern of investigators evaluating the intracavitary approach to the treatment of tumors confined to body cavities is that of the potential compromise of therapeutic efficacy due to decreased drug delivery by capillary flow. While it is not possible to directly measure the amount of drug reaching the tumor by direct penetration from the instilled agent or from systemic delivery of absorbed drug, several general comments related to this issue can be made.

First, because of its unique intrinsic fluorescence, Ozols et al. were able to monitor the penetration of doxorubicin in a mouse transplantable ovarian cancer model (8). Following intraperitoneal administration of this agent, bright doxorubicin-specific intranuclear fluorescence was demonstrated only in the outermost four to six cell layers of tumor. Unexpectedly, after intravenous treatment, faint fluorescence was observed in a patchy distribution throughout the tumor. However, in spite of the apparently limited penetrability of doxorubicin in this animal model, the efficacy of intraperitoneal drug administration was quite dramatic. While 70% of mice receiving a single intraperitoneal 10% lethal dose of doxorubicin (5 mg/kg) experienced long-term survival (>60 days) when given 10^6 tumor cells, there were no long-term survivors among mice administered doxorubicin intravenously with a comparable 10% lethal dose of the drug. Thus, at least in this model system, the efficacy of therapy was not clearly related to the observed level of penetration of drug into tumor, and cure was achieved only during treatment by the intraperitoneal route.

Perhaps most importantly, however, the issue of decreased drug delivery by capillary flow becomes moot if it becomes possible to deliver as much drug systemically when the agent is administered intrapleurally or intraperitoneally as when the drug is infused intravenously at maximally tolerated dosages. If this condition can be satisfied, then any contribution to efficacy of treatment of tumor in direct contact with the drug will be <u>additive</u> to the effects of the systemically delivered drug. While the major benefit of such treatment would clearly be on free-floating tumor cells (in ascites, pleural fluid) or small tumor nodules, even large tumor masses might be influenced by the direct penetration of the drug onto surfaces exposed to chemotherapy- containing fluid. For example, as discussed in another paper in this symposium, while at maximally tolerated dosages of intraperitoneally administered cisplatin (270 mg/m^2) with the simultaneous intravenous administration of sodium thiosulfate, the area under the peritoneal cavity elimination curve averaged 12-fold higher than the area under the plasma curve; the area under the concentration curve for the plasma <u>increased</u> twofold compared to that for cisplatin administered intravenously at a dose of 100 mg/m^2 (6).

The use of sodium thiosulfate with cisplatin to neutralize the toxic effects of this agent on the kidneys highlights a major potential advantage of the intracavitary approach to the treatment of tumors localized to body cavities. The ability to neutralize the toxic (and potentially therapeutic) effects of chemotherapeutic agents prior or subsequent to their entrance into the systemic circulation while allowing high concentrations of active drug to be delivered in close proximity to the tumor will hopefully increase tumor cell kill while reducing normal tissue damage. An example of neutralization of a chemotherapeutic agent prior to its entrance into the systemic circulation is that of the hepatic deamination of cytarabine during intraperitonel administration (9). The use of sodium thiosulfate along with cisplatin demonstrates the efficacy of a systemically administered neutralizing agent (6).

Another issue raised by the intracavitary administration of chemotherapeutic agents is that of local toxicity, particularly the development of chemical peritonitis. Experience with intraperitoneally administered vinblastine emphasizes this point (10). Two patients treated with this agent in a phase I trial developed an adynamic ileus following treatment, with one patient requiring surgery because of this problem. An additional example is that of the intraperitoneal administration of doxorubicin. In our experience, this agent, when administered at a concentration of 18 μM (20 mg/2 liter treatment volume) in combination with cisplatin and cytarabine, has been associated with an unacceptable level of abdominal pain, with 60% of patients requiring narcotic analgesia or having pain lasting longer than 72 hours. Also, while others have demonstrated that this agent can be administered with acceptable local toxicity, pain remains the dose-limiting toxicity (11).

There is the additional concern that even if local pain is not excessive with intracavitary drug administration, a sub-clinical inflammatory reaction may result in adhesion formation, leading to bowel obstruction or interference with adequate drug distribution during future courses. Careful evaluation of both immediate and long-term effects on patients treated with various intracavitary regimens will be necessary to fully characterize the unique toxicities of this treatment approach. It must also be appreciated, however, that certain effects of therapy may be more related to efficacy than to toxicity of treatment. For example, it is possible that dead and dying tumor may become necrotic and cause bowel perforation or that a non-specific inflammatory response may actually promote tumor cell kill.

The placement of a semi-permanent catheter into the body cavity to be treated during intracavitary chemotherapy administration is essential to provide safe, long-term access. Therefore, there exists the continuous risk of bacterial infection each time the catheter is manipulated. While it is clearly possible to treat patients intraperitoneally or intrapleurally by the percutaneous placement of a paracentesis or thoracentesis catheter _in the presence of ascites or pleural fluid,_ there is a significant risk of bowel perforation or pneumothorax with repeated use of these procedures. In addition, in responding patients, the amount of fluid present will likely decrease, markedly increasing the hazards associated with blind catheter placement.

Much has been learned about long-term catheter safety and care from the experience with continuous peritoneal dialysis for renal insufficiency (12-13). Unfortunately, infection of catheters remains a common problem (13-14). Due to their normal presence on skin, the most common pathogens to cause catheter infections in this clinical setting have been _Staphlococcus aureus_ and _Staphlococcus epidermidis_. In our experience _Staphlococcus epidermidis_ has been the major cause of catheter-related peritoneal infections. Unfortunately, while this organism is usually sensitive _in vitro_ to several antimicrobial agents, removal of the catheter is frequently required to cure the infection. In addition, experience with the immunocompromised host who develops a _Staphlococcus epidermidis_ infection has suggested that in spite of _in vitro_ sensitivity of the organism to cephalosporins, these agents are frequently unable to erradicate the infection, particularly in the continued presence of a foreign body (15). Vancomycin has been demonstrated to be extremely effective in treating _Staphlococcus epidermidis_ peritoneal infections in the dialysis population and to successfully treat this infection in immunocompromised patients failing cephalosporin therapy (14-15). In our experience, several patients have failed treatment for bacterial peritonitis caused by _Staphlococcus epidermidis_ when cephalosporins were administered but responded sucessfully when vancomycin therapy was instituted.

It is unknown at present whether or not the institution of completely subcutaneous infusion systems (described in detail in another report in this symposium) will significantly reduce the incidence of catheter-related infection. However, they have clearly improved patient acceptance of intracavitary therapy and have significantly reduced the need for patient maintenance of the catheter with its inherent risk of introduction of infection. It should be pointed out here that there is one major difference between the currently utilized subcutaneous infusion systems and the standard Tenckhoff catheters used for chronic peritoneal dialysis. Using the standard Tenckhoff, it is possible to administer a two liter treatment volume in 10-15 minutes, while the subcutaneous system generally requires 40-70 minutes to deliver the same amount of fluid.

The optimal drugs, dosages and treatment schedules for the different malignancies involving various body cavities remain to be defined. The tremendous pharmacokinetic advantage achievable during intracavitary therapy allows one to potentially deliver cytotoxic concentrations of drug into body cavities with non-toxic levels reaching the systemic circulation. Thus, for the first time, one has the potential of rationally administering cell-cycle phase-specific agents (such as cytarabine) for weeks or even months to solid tumors principally localized to body cavities (ovarian carcinoma, mesothelioma). Unfortunately, while this concept has great appeal, the practical issue of developing a safe and economical delivery system remains formidable.

Finally, as regards the potential of combination intracavitary chemotherapy, while two drugs may be safe and effective when administered individually by the intracavitary route,the combination of the two agents may result in new and excessive toxicities. It is only through well-designed and carefully conducted clinical trials that the safety and effectiveness of this innovative form of therapy can be evaluated. The eventual role of such therapy in patients with malignant disease refractory to front-line chemotherapy or as initial treatment cannot be defined until the questions addressed in this paper have been answered. In addition, in the future, controlled trials comparing intracavitary therapy with standard treatment programs for the different tumors being evaluated will need to be conducted.

REFERENCES

1. Dedrick RL, Myers CE, Bungay PM, DeVita VT Jr: Pharmacokinetic rationale for peritoneal administration in the treatment of ovarian cancer. Cancer Treat Rep 62:1-9, 1978.
2. Katz ME, Schwartz PE, Kapp DS, Luikart S: Epithelial carcinoma of the ovary: current strategies. Ann Intern Med 95:98-111, 1981.
3. Rosenshein N, Blake D, McIntyre PA, Parmley T, Natarajan TK, Dvornicky J, Nickoloff E: The effect of volume on the distribution of substances instilled into the peritoneal cavity. Gynecologic Oncol 6:106-110, 1978.
4. Tully TE, Goldberg ME, Loken MK: The use of ^{99m}Tc-sulfur colloid to assess the distribution of ^{32}P chromic phosphate. J Nucl Med 15:190-191, 1974.
5. Taylor A Jr: Loculation as a contraindication to intracavitary ^{32}P chromic phosphate therapy. J Nucl Med 16:318-319, 1975.
6. Howell SB, Pfeifle CE, Wung WE, Olshen RA, Lucas WE, Yon JL, Green MR: Intraperitoneal cisplatin with systemic thiosulfate protection. Ann Intern Med 97:845-851, 1982.
7. Dunnick NR, Jones RB, Doppman JL, Speyer J, Myers CE: Intraperitoneal contrast infusion for assessment of intraperitoneal fluid dynamics. AJR 133:221-223, 1979.
8. Ozols RF, Locker GY, Doroshow JH, Grotzinger KR, Myers CE, Young RC: Pharmacokinetics of adriamycin and tissue penetration in murine ovarian cancer. Cancer Res 39:3209-3214, 1979.
9. King ME, Howell SB: Intraperitoneal cytarabine therapy in ovarian carcinoma. J Clin Oncol (in press), 1983.
10. Alberts DS, Chen HSG, Chang SY, Peng YM: The disposition of intraperitoneal bleomycin, melphalan, and vinblastine in cancer patients. Recent Results in Cancer Res 74:293-299, 1980.
11. Ozols RF, Young RC, Speyer JL, Sugarbaker PH, Green R, Jenkins J, Myers CE: Phase I and pharmacological studies of adriamycin administered intraperitoneally to patients with ovarian cancer. Cancer 42:4265-4269, 1982.

12. Gloor HJ, Nichols WK, Sorkin MI, Prowant BF, Kennedy JM, Baker B, Nolph KD: Peritoneal access and related complications in continuous ambulatory peritoneal dialysis. Am J Med 74:593-598, 1983.

13. Rubin J, Rogers WA, Taylor HM, Everett ED, Prowant BF, Fruto LV, Nolph KD: Peritonitis during continuous ambulatory peritoneal dialysis. Ann Intern Med 92:7-13, 1980.

14. Krothapalli RK, Senekjian HD, Ayus JC: Efficacy of intravenous vancomycin in the treatment of gram-positive peritonitis in long-term peritoneal dialysis. Am J Med 75:345-348, 1983.

15. Wade JC, Schimpff SC, Newman KA, Wiernik PH: *Staphlococcus epidermidis*: an increasing cause of infection in patients with granulocytopenia. Ann Intern Med 97:503-508, 1982.

INTRA-ARTERIAL THERAPY OF HEPATIC METASTASES

WILLIAM D. ENSMINGER, PH.D., M.D.,

INTRODUCTION

There are several unique aspects of hepatic arterial chemotherapy, making it a treatment modality that is both rational and of great therapeutic potential (Table 1). Recent developments have defined the prerequisites for successful hepatic arterial chemotherapy and provided the methods for achieving those prerequisites (Table 2)[1,2]. The development of the totally implanted drug delivery system, its successful application in several large phase II studies in colorectal liver metastases, and the FDA approval for commercial sale of the Model 400 Infusaid pump (Infusaid Corp., Norwood, MA) have provided a major impetus to the entire field of regional chemotherapy. The phase II studies of note are from the University of Michigan and the University of Alabama, and both have been recently published in detail[3, 4]. Thus, this discussion will only summarize these results and describe the problems in their interpretation and in performing the essential randomized phase III studies.

Table 1. Unique Aspects of Hepatic Arterial Chemotherapy

A. Extensive hepatic drug metabolism/extraction for drugs (FU and FUDR) of greatest current utility.

B. Dual blood supply to liver with dependence of tumor primarily on hepatic artery for nutrient flow.

C. Relatively high drug tolerance of liver
   1. Cytokinetically inactive
   2. Excess functional capacity
   3. Regenerative potential

D. Frequently applicable in metastatic disease.

Table 2. Prerequisites for Successful Hepatic Arterial Chemotherapy

A. Correct drug:
   1. Appropriate degree of antitumor activity to generate benefit from dose-response effects
   2. Usual dose-limiting toxicities extrahepatic
   3. Appropriate pharmacokinetic properties:
      a. High total body clearance (essential)
      b. Extracted by liver (important, but not essential)
      c. Extrahepatic clearance also present

B. Access to tumor arterial supply complete and reliable:
   1. Usually need to infuse entire liver
   2. Catheter cannot move about nor can it generate thrombosis/vascular injury
   3. Need to monitor infusion pattern
      a. Role for Tc-MAA nuclide angiography
      b. Flow rate dependence of infusion
      c. Potential development of thrombosis/collaterals with loss of complete infusion pattern

C. Reliable device for controlled rate infusion:

1. External pumps
2. Implantable Model 400 Infusaid pump

PHASE II STUDIES

The Phase II study at the University of Michigan was initiated approximately four years ago(3). The study group consisted of 93 evaluabale patients, 50 of whom had metastatic colorectal cancer confined to the liver and 43 of whom had hepatic plus extrahepatic metastatic disease. Patients with liver only metastatic disease received 0.3 mg/kg/day of fluorodeoxyuridine (FUDR) for two weeks alternating with 2 weeks of saline. Patients with extrahepatic disease initially, or in whom it developed, and those failing FUDR all received in addition, mitomycin C, 15 mg/M^2, every 6-8 weeks through the pump sideport. Table 3 summarizes the therapeutic results achieved in this study. Responses were defined either by liver scan or physical examination. Essentially all patients who have died did so due to progressive extrahepatic disease, indicating that regional hepatic tumor control had been achieved. This is in contrast with other studies which indicate that progressive regional hepatic cancer is the usual cause of death in such a patient population(5). Toxicities (Table 4) were not inconsequential and included symptoms of gastritis in 56% of patients and chemical hepatitis in 56% of patients. Cholecystitis requiring cholecystectomy occurred in 3% of patients, and sclerosing cholangitis, which was not reversible, in 1% of patients. It is felt that the actual incidence of cholecystitis is larger than noted and that some of the symptoms attributed to gastritis were due to chronic cholecystitis. For that reason, we and others are currently performing cholecystectomy routinely at time of catheter and pump implant.

Table 3. Summary of Therapeutic Results With Hepatic Arterial Chemotherapy for Colorectal Liver Metastases

	Resp.	Stable	Prog.	Median Duration Resp. (Mo)	Median Survival[b] (Mo)	Alive[c] (2/84)
Liver only (50 pts)	83%	12%	5%	13[a]	18 (25)	6 (12%)
Liver plus (43 pts)	74%	16%	9%	6	9 (14)	2 (5%)

[a]The median duration of response to FUDR alone was 7 months.
[b]From pump implant (From time of diagnosis of liver metastases).
[c]All beyond 3 years from implantation.

Table 4. Toxicities With (Protracted) Treatment With FUDR (and Mitomycin):

A. Common (50% of patients)
   1. Gastritis and ulcers--related to drug, dose, schedule, duration, ischemia, stress, unligated or reformed extrahepatic vessels.
   2. Hepatitis--related to drug, dose, schedule, duration, pre-existing or recent bout of hepatitis.

B. Uncommon (<5% of patients)
   1. Sclerosing cholangitis--biliary tree blood supply primarily arterial, not portal; chronic process
   2. Myelosuppression--Prior radiotherapy, active infection

The phase II evaluation at the University of Alabama[4] developed out of the program at the University of Michigan and used the same method of drug delivery system implantation with TcMAA to monitor complete hepatic infusion and a similar treatment regimen. The response rate denoted by a fall in carcinoembryonic antigen level by onethird was 88%, and compared to matched historical controls, treated patients lived 12 to 18 months longer. Another recent study by Weiss et al.[6] of 17 patients contrasts with these results, showing only 5 responses by CT scan. It is noteworthy that these latter investigators only achieved drug infusion to the entire liver, as monitored by Tc 99-macroaggregated nuclide angiography, in 62% of patients. In the studies at Michigan and Alabama, complete hepatic infusional coverage was achieved in all patients.

CONCLUSION

Phase II studies are not a "gold standard" for efficacy, and only randomized phase III studies can control for such important factors as patient selection and method of response evaluation. To this end, a consortium of five institutions has joined together to form the Hepatic Tumor Study Group. A randomized phase III study has recently been initiated by this group to examine the impact of hepatic arterial and combined hepatic arterial/systemic chemotherapy on the survival of patients with colorectal cancer confined to the liver at time of implantation of the infusion system. This study and the others described in this symposium are in difficulty due to low patient accrual arising out of widespread commercialization of the Infusaid system. Unfortunately, a portion of those implanting the Infusaid system will not have the patient volume, investigative tendencies, or commitment necessary to carry on a program which benefits most patients. Despite these problems, one can hope that the revitalization of interest in hepatic arterial chemotherapy will be more meaningfully sustained than was the initial introduction of this modality in the early 1960's.

REFERENCES

1. Ensminger W, Niederhuber J, Dakhil S, Thrall J, Wheeler R: Totally implanted drug delivery system for hepatic arterial chemotherapy. Cancer Treat Rep (65):393-400, 1981.
2. Ensminger WD, Gyves JW: Regional cancer chemotherapy. Cancer Treat Rep (68):101-115, 1984.
3. Niederhuber JE, Ensminger WD, Gyves JW, Thrall J, Walker S, Cozzi E: Regional chemotherapy of colorectal cancer metastatic to the liver. Cancer (53):1336-1343, 1984.
4. Balch CM, Urist MM, Soong SJ, McGregor M: A prospective phase II clinical trial of continuous FUDR regional chemotherapy for colorectal metastases to the liver using a totally implantable drug infusion pump. Ann Surg (198):567-573, 1983.
5. Goslin R, Steele G, Zamcheck N, Mayer R, MacIntyre J: Factors influencing survival in patients with hepatic metastases from adenocarcinoma of the colon or rectum. Dis Col & Rect (25):749-754, 1982.
6. Weiss GR, Garnick MB, Osteen RT, Steele GD, Wilson RE, Schade D, Kaplan WD, Boxt LM, Kandarpa K, Mayer RJ, Frei ET, III: Long-term hepatic arterial infusion of 5-fluorodeoxyuridine for liver metastases using an implantable infusion pump. J Clin Oncol (1):337-343, 1983.

INTRA-ARTERIAL VS INTRAVENOUS FUDR FOR COLORECTAL CANCER METASTATIC TO THE LIVER: A NORTHERN CALIFORNIA ONCOLOGY GROUP STUDY

B.J. LEWIS, M.D., R.J. STAGG, PHARM.D., M.A. FRIEDMAN, M.D., R.J. IGNOFFO, PHARM.D., AND D.C. HOHN, M.D.

1. INTRODUCTION

Conventional management of hepatic metastases from colorectal cancer has been a frustrating endeavor. Systemic chemotherapy, hepatic radiation, and hepatic arterial embolization or ligation have low response rates; few patients are eligible for partial hepatectomy to eradicate anatomically limited disease; and the role of liver-directed therapy with drugs in patients with metastases confined to the liver remains uncertain.

The rationale for liver-directed treatment arises from several elements. First, liver metastases derive their nutrient blood supply primarily from the hepatic artery, while hepatocytes are predominantly supplied by the portal venous system. Consequently, the concentration of drugs given directly into the hepatic artery will be higher for tumor cells than for hepatocytes. The drug level will also be high in comparison to drug administered IV, because the compound has not been diluted by the total blood volume. Second, when a drug is highly extracted by the liver, systemic drug levels will be lower with hepatic artery infusion (HAI) than with IV drugs. Hence, toxicity in target organs such as the bone marrow and gut should be diminished with HAI.

Over the last two decades, there has been a wide experience with HAI, mostly using the fluoropyrimidines, 5-fluorouracil and FUDR. These studies, summarized in a recent review (1), suggest that HAI may be better than IV administration in terms of overall response rate, in producing responses in patients with disease refractory to IV 5FU, and in lessening or shifting the forms of toxicity. However, problems in study design do not allow definitive conclusions about whether HAI is truly more effective and worth the added effort.

Until recently, the technology of HAI has been a limiting factor. Percutaneous arterial catheters have a limited life and a high complication rate (2), allowing relatively brief periods of drug delivery. For cycle active agents such as the fluoropyrimidines, where repeated cycles of prolonged, continuous drug exposure may increase tumor cell kill, this limitation is of particular concern (3).

The advent of implanted infusion pumps has greatly increased the feasibility of prolonged drug delivery by HAI (4). While pump placement requires a laparotomy, the operation enables the surgeon to assess resectability and to achieve a complete perfusion even in the presence of anomalous hepatic arterial anatomy. Arterial feeders to the stomach and duodenum can be ligated to prevent drug damage to these organs. Intraoperatively, use of fluorescein injection into the catheter and a Wood's light confirms perfusion of the entire liver and the absence of extrahepatic perfusion. Since the system is totally implanted, it greatly increases the duration of HAI and lessens the complications of arterial thrombosis, catheter migration, infection, and bleeding. Patients do not have to contend with an external device which could inhibit daily activities or freedom of movement. Most importantly, Ensminger and colleagues (4), as reviewed elsewhere in this conference, and other workers (5-8) have reported increased antitumor activity with HAI of FUDR using the implanted pump.

However, because the hepatic extraction of FUDR when given IV is also high (80% versus 95% when given by HAI), the question arose whether IV administration of the drug might be as effective as HAI for treating colorectal cancer metastatic to the liver. IV pumps could be placed under local anesthesia without hospitalization, avoiding the need for laparatomy and the problems posed by hepatic arterial anomalies. To address this issue, in 1982 Drs. Hohn and Friedman, in conjunction with the Northern California Oncology Group, began development of a randomized comparison of FUDR therapy by continuous infusion either IV or via HAI.

2. PROCEDURE

2.1. Patient Selection

Entry criteria for the study include informed consent, histologic diagnosis of the primary lesion, and liver metastases demonstrated by CAT scan or surgical exploration. The Karnofsky performance has to be $>$ 50% and allowable prior therapy is limited to $<$ 10 grams cumulative dose of IV 5FU or pelvic radiation for the adjuvant therapy of resected rectal cancer. Patients also must have adequate hematologic, renal, and hepatic function (no prior liver irradiation, prothrombin time $<$ 15 seconds, no gross ascites, bilirubin $<$ 7, and no encephalopathy).

Extrahepatic disease is excluded with physical examination, chest x-ray and abdominal/pelvic CAT scan. Patients are stratified according to KPS (50-60%, 70-80%, 90-100%), bilirubin ($<$ 2 mgm%, $>$ 2 mgm%), and amount of liver replacement (minor (10% or less) ; moderate (10-30%) ; massive (30+%)) as visualized on CAT scan or direct inspection.

.2. IA Therapy

Patients randomized to IA therapy receive a preoperative celiac angiogram to define the arterial anatomy of the liver. Patients with potentially resectable lesions undergo laparotomy with intraoperative randomization if unresectable. In patients receiving HAI, the gastroduodenal artery is ligated and the catheter placed at the junction of the gastroduodenal artery and hepatic artery. Arterial branches to the stomach or duodenum beyond this point are ligated. An intraoperative fluorescein injection is used to confirm bilobar perfusion and absence of flow to the gut. An Infusaid pump is placed in a pocket in the abdominal wall and filled with heparinized bacteriostatic water. Postoperatively, technetium 99 macro-aggregated albumin scans are used to further confirm the adequacy of the perfusion. FUDR therapy is instituted on the fourth or fifth postoperative day.

.3. IV Therapy

The pump is placed into a subcutaneous pocket in the pectoral area and the catheter passed into the superior vena cava via the cephalic vein or the transected proximal stump of the external jugular vein. Catheter position is verified radiographically. The pump is loaded intraoperatively with warm water containing heparin and FUDR.

.4. Drug Treatment

IA patients begin therapy at 0.2 mg/kg/day for 14 days per cycle with intervening 14 day periods when the pump is filled with heparinized water (Initially, the starting dose was 0.3 mg /kg/day, but because of untoward toxicity (biliary sclerosis) this dose was reduced. (See below.). If the serum alkaline phosphatase doubles, FUDR is withheld until the value returns to baseline. If the value triples, the patient is evaluated with cholangiography for bile duct sclerosis (once disease progression is excluded).

IV patients start at 0.05 mg /kg/day for 14 days per cycle as above with escalation of the dose by 0.025 mg /kg/day per cycle until a maximum of 0.15 mg /kg/day is reached or until toxicity (diarrhea) appears. At the point of toxicity, the last preceding dose level is used for subsequent cycles, and therapy is not reinstituted until side effects have abated. If gastrointestinal toxicity appears during the 14 days of the drug cycle, the pump is immediately unloaded and filled with heparinized water.

2.5. Tracking Studies and Measurement of Effect

Liver function tests are obtained every two weeks in the IA group and monthly in the IV group. In both arms of the trial, hematology studies are drawn every 6 weeks and CEA levels every 2 months. CAT scans are performed after every third drug cycle. Chest x-rays are obtained every two months.

A complete response is defined as a return of CAT scan, CEA, liver function tests, and liver size to normal. A partial response requires a 50% decrease in the size (product of the longest perpendicular diameters) or measurable lesions on CAT scan. The stable disease designation indicates non-progression and non-response. Two cycles of therapy are required before a patient is said to have progressive disease. Time to progression is measured from the date of randomization.

3. RESULTS

3.1. Patient Characteristics

To date, 55 patients have been randomized: 26 to IA therapy, 29 to IV treatment. Five patients in the IA group were not treated. In 2 patients this was because extrahepatic disease was discovered at the time of laparotom for catheter placement. One patient refused therapy, and 2 patients were inappropriately randomized because of either extrahepatic disease or too low a performance status. Two patients in the IV group were randomized but then withdrew from the study. Thus, 21 patients have begun IA therapy; 27 IV therapy, and,to date,16 and 17 patients respectively in each group are evaluable for toxicity and response. The median time on study is 6 months for IA patients, 6 months for IV patients, and the median number of drug cycles is 3 for the IA and 7 for the IV therapy group.

3.2. Response to Treatment

3.2.1. IA Therapy. One of 16 (6%) patients had a complete response

(CR); 6 of 16 (38%) had a partial response (PR), and 4 (25%) have had stable disease (SD). Five of 16 (31%) had progressive disease (PD). Median duration of response was 4.5 months. To date, 13 patients have progressed; 5 in the liver, 4 only outside the liver, and 4 both in and outside the liver. Median times to progression for each of these groups were 3, 4, and 7.5 months respectively. Six patients have died.

3.2.3. IV Therapy. One of 17 patients had a CR (6%); 4 of 17 (24%) had a PR; 8 of 17 (47%) had SD; and 4 of 17 (24%) had PD. Median duration of response was 6 months. To date, 12 patients have progressed; 6 in the liver only, 1 outside the liver, and 5 both in and outside the liver. Median times to progression were 6, 5, and 6 months respectively. Three patients have died.

3.3. Toxicity

The median tolerated doses were 0.065 mg /kg/day in the IA group and 0.09 mg /kg/day in the IV group. In the IA arm of the trial, all 16 patients developed toxicity manifested by cyclic increases in alkaline phosphatase (and, in some, bilirubin levels) which did not reflect disease progression. In 7 patients, bile duct sclerosis (BDS) was documented by cholangiography and by histologic analysis of liver biopsies. In 5 patients, IA therapy had to be terminated because of this complication. Nine patients had pump pocket seromas, and no patients had pump pocket infections. Three patients required cholecystectomy for drug-induced acalculous cholecystitis.

In the IV arm of the study, all 17 patients developed diarrhea as the limiting toxicity. One patient each had a photosensitivity reaction, Herpes zoster infection, anorexia, and nausea and vomiting. No IV patient required treatment termination due to toxicity. There was 1 pump pocket seroma and 1 pump pocket infection.

3.4. Economics

At UCSF, start up costs are approximately $10,000 for IA pump placement (staging studies, angiography, radionuclide perfusion study, hospitalization, operating room and anesthesia charges, pump purchase and professional fees). For IV therapy, the cost is $4,000 to $5,000 (staging studies, outpatient surgery charges, pump purchase, and professional fee). The costs for pump maintenance are the same for each arm. Expenses related to toxicity were high in the IA arm (hospitalization, cholecystectomy, cholangiography) and were minimal in the IV arm.

4. DISCUSSION

The study accrued a number of patients while in a pilot phase and was activated as a formal NCOG study in April, 1983. In the last six months, we have seen a fall-off in patient accession. We assume this is due to the increasing *ad hoc* use of the pump by community physicians who, in effect, are assuming that IA FUDR therapy is established therapy for metastatic liver lesions.

While our patient numbers are still small, the data suggests that IA therapy with FUDR is less effective than previously reported and that continuous IV treatment is of comparable potency but is less toxic, less cumbersome, and less expensive. More patients and more observation time will be required to determine the comparative benefits of these therapies and to fully assess the impact of these treatments upon survival and the natural history of metastatic colorectal cancer.

Patients on IA therapy initially received FUDR at 0.3 mg/kg/day. Because of the frequency of BDS, we have decreased the starting dose to 0.2 mg/kg/day and still anticipate that dose de-escalation may be necessary in the majority of patients. IV patients begin at 0.05 mg/kg/day with escalation to toxicity. Consequently, the patients in the IA arm have received a *lower* cumulative dose of FUDR than the patients in the IV arm. Given the high hepatic extraction of the drug by either route, and the high incidence of toxic side effects with IA infusion, the "advantage" of the high local FUDR concentration achieved with HAI may well be a disadvantage. BDS in fact may be a direct consequence of high local FUDR concentration in the arterial supply. It is interesting to note that the sclerotic lesions anatomically correspond to areas where the common bile duct receives its arterial supply from the hepatic artery (9). We have also seen an apparent correlation between clinical responses and the development of BDS. All of our patients with BDS had either a PR or, in one case, a CR to treatment. It is intriguing to speculate that the same biochemical vulnerability to the drug is present in the tumor and in normal bile duct. Another group has also observed this relationship (Bernard Levin, personal communication).

Attention to eliminating arterial drainage of FUDR outside the hepatic artery circuit at the time of laparotomy appears to have prevented the mucosal toxicity in the stomach and duodenum seen in earlier trials (10). Although we are not routinely endoscoping patients to visualize changes in the gastroduodenal mucosa (Bernard Levin, personal communication), there have been no patients with clinical symptoms and signs of ulcer or gastritis in our series.

The relative costs of the two routes of delivery are obvious. HAI is more expensive than IV therapy in actual terms because of the need for laparotomy, hospitalization, and added diagnostic studies, and in potential terms because of costs associated with biliary toxicity.

We continue to emphasize the importance of careful and systematic documentation of response. We do not regard changes in radionuclide scans or changes in blood tests as "hard" response criteria, and we use CAT scans as the final indicator of response.

Interpretation and management are more difficult when a patient who has stable or responding tumor in the liver progresses extrahepatically. It has been our practice to continue FUDR therapy in spite of extrahepatic disease until there is progression in the liver or until the extrahepatic disease (or the patient) demands additional treatment. In 3 cases, when patients have had hepatic progression on IV FUDR, changing the pump to provide HAI has produced transient responses. The numbers,however, are too small to allow further comment. Since variations in "post-pump" treatments and the therapeutic response to them may differentially affect overall survival, this parameter may be particularly difficult to compare between the IA and IV arms of the study.

Finally, we think the results and trends to date strongly underscore the need to complete this and similar randomized trials. We urge community physicians to enter eligible patients into formal studies so that the overall impact of FUDR infusion and the implantable pump technology can be defined.

5. REFERENCES

1. Stagg, RJ, Lewis BJ, Friedman MA, Ignoffo RJ, Hohn DC: Hepatic arterial chemotherapy for colorectal cancer metastatic to the liver. Ann Intern Med (100): 1984 (In Press).
2. Oberfield RA, McCaffrey JA, Polio J, Clouse ME, Hamilton T: Prolonged and continuous percutaneous intra-arterial hepatic

infusion chemotherapy in advanced metastatic liver adenocarcinoma from colorectal primary. Cancer (44): 414-423, 1979.

3. Shackney SE, Ritch PS: Cell kinetics. In: Chabner B (ed) Pharmacologic principles of cancer treatment. W.B. Saunders Co., Philadelphia, 1982, pp 45-76.
4. Ensminger W, Niederhuber J, Gyves J, Thrall J, Cozzi E, Doan K: Effective control of liver metastases from colon cancer with an implanted system for hepatic arterial chemotherapy. Proc Am Soc Clin Oncol (1): 94, 1982.
5. Wiess GR, Garnick MB, Osteen RT, Steele GD Jr, Wilson RE, Schade D, Kaplan WD, Boxt LM, Kandarpa K, Mayer RJ, Frei ET III: Long-term hepatic arterial infusion of 5-fluorodeoxyuridine for liver metastases using an implantable infusion pump. J Clin Oncol (1): 337-344, 1983.
6. Kemeny N, Daly JM, Olderman P, Shike M: Hepatic infusion chemotherapy for metastatic colorectal carcinoma, results and complications. Proc Am Soc Clin Oncol (2): 123, 1983.
7. Balch CM, Urist MM, Soong SJ, McGregor ML: A prospective phase II clinical trial of continuous FUDR regional chemotherapy for colorectal metastases to the liver using a totally implantable drug infusion pump. Ann of Surg (198): 567-573, 1983.
8. Levin B, Karl R, Dubrow R, Cooper M, Hagle M, Cooper R: Regional hepatic chemotherapy for metastatic cancer with an implantable drug infusion system. Clin Res (30): 783A, 1983.
9. Northover JA, Terblinche J: A new look at the arterial supply of the bile duct in man and its surgical implications. Br J Surg (66): 379-384, 1979.
10. Hohn D, Stagg R, Ignoffo RJ, Friedman MA, Melnick J, Altman D, Lewis B: Incidence and prevention of complications of cyclic hepatic artery infusions (HAI) of floxuridine (FUDR): Severe biliary sclerosis, gastritis and ulcer. Proc Am Soc Clin Oncol (3): 1984 (Submitted).

RANDOMIZED STUDY OF INTRAHEPATIC VS SYSTEMIC INFUSION OF FLUORODEOXYURIDINE IN PATIENTS WITH LIVER METASTASES FROM COLORECTAL CARCINOMA (PRELIMINARY RESULTS).

N. KEMENY, J. DALY, H. CHUN, P. ODERMAN, G. PETRONI, AND N. GELLER

Hepatic metastases represent a common site of dissemination for a number of primary malignancies, especially gastrointestinal neoplasms. Sixty percent of patients with colorectal carcinoma develop liver metastases during the course of their illness,[1] and 30% will have hepatic metastases as the only site of disease.[2] The average response rate of metastatic colon cancer to traditional bolus 5-FU is around 20%.[3] The response rate is approximately the same even if patients with liver metastases are considered alone. While the addition of MeCCNU to 5-FU did not increase the response rate for the total population or for those with liver metastases, the combination of MeCCNU, 5-FU, Vincristine and Streptozotocin (MOF-Strep) increased the response rate for both groups up to around 30%.[3]

Although the liver has a dual blood supply, it has been suggested that hepatic tumors derive their blood supply primarily from the hepatic artery.[4] Thus, an infusion of chemotherapeutic agents via the hepatic artery may provide a high drug concentration directly to the tumor and spare the normal liver tissue which receives the blood primarily via the portal vein. It has also been suggested that certain drugs, such as 5-Fluoro-2-deoxyuridine (FUDR), have a higher hepatic extraction, thus resulting in lower systemic exposure and perhaps in a higher local drug concentration.[5]

Earlier trials with hepatic artery perfusion used an external pump which required hospitalization and/or patient immobilization. Because of the hindrance to normal activity, few oncologists advocated the use of hepatic artery perfusion despite the apparently higher response rates. Development of a totally

Table 1. Result of Hepatic Artery Infusion via Infusaid Pump.

	Number of Patients	% Response
Ensminger	60	83
Balch	50	83
Barone	18	56
Cohen	26	53
Kemeny	41	41
Johnson	17	36
Levin	31	30
Weiss	17	29

implantable infusion device provided a new stimulus for the infusion advocates. Although an impressive 83% response rate was reported in the first study with continuous FUDR infusion via the hepatic artery using the infusaid pump,[6] most of the other investigators using this method could not reproduce such a high response rate (Table 1).[7] Nevertheless, the mean response rate of 59% is still higher than the mean response rate with systemic chemotherapy trials.

Although surgical and technical complications with the use of an implantable pump have been minimal, chemotherapy-related complications have been substantial. In a study at Memorial Sloan-Kettering Cancer Center (MSKCC) on 45 patients,[7] 30% had endoscopically documented gastrointestinal ulceration. If severe gastritis and duodenitis are included, 50% had significant gastrointestinal disease. Hepatic toxicity was also frequently seen; an elevation of serum bilirubin level above 3 mg/dl was observed in 20% of the patients, and an elevation of SGOT level in 65%. Two patients developed strictures of their bile duct resembling sclerosing cholangitis.[7]

Another problem with intrahepatic therapy is the possibility of developing extrahepatic disease, since only the liver is being treated. At MSKCC, 13 of 41 adequately treated patients developed extrahepatic disease.[7] In a study by Cady and Oberfield,[8] 59% of the responders to intrahepatic therapy died with extrahepatic disease.

It is difficult to interpret the true impact of hepatic infusion therapy on response and survival without a prospective randomized trial comparing it to systemic infusion therapy. In such a study, patients would need to be stratified for parameters known to influence the response rate and survival, such as performance status (PS), percent liver involvement and initial lactic dehydrogenase (LDH) level. Patients with poor PS usually are not included in many of the hepatic infusion trials because of the requirement of an exploratory laparotomy. Instead, these same patients with poor PS are entered into systemic chemotherapy trials.

In a study at MSKCC on 220 patients with advanced metastatic colorectal carcinoma, the most significant factor affecting the survival and response was the initial LDH level.[9] Patients with normal initial LDH and carcinoembryonic antigen (CEA) levels had a median survival of 32 months versus only 8 months for those with abnormal initial LDH and CEA values. It has also been reported by many investigators that the extent of liver involvement by tumor is an independent prognostic factor influencing survival (Table 2). Therefore, the true difference between intrahepatic and systemic chemotherapy can only be shown by a concurrent randomized study.

A prospective randomized study is in progress at MSKCC which will compare intrahepatic infusion to systemic infusion applying the same chemotherapeutic agent (FUDR), schedule and method of administration. Patients with measurable, metastatic colorectal carcinoma to the liver without extrahepatic disease are eligible. Patients with a Karnofsky PS less than 60% and a serum bilirubin greater than 4.0 mg/dl are excluded.

After stratification by LDH level ($<$300 U/l vs $\geq$300 U/l) and percent liver involvement ($<$50% vs $\geq$50%), all patients are randomized to either intrahepatic or systemic therapy prior to surgery. The extent of liver involvement is assessed medically by an evaluation of computerized tomography (CTT) and/or radionuclide liver scans. The information is placed in a sealed envelope and only opened after the extent of liver involvement

Table 2. Influence of the Extent of Liver Involvement by Tumor on Survival.

References	Liver Involvement	Survival (months)*
Kemeny[7]	20%	13
	21-40%	13
	41-60%	11
	61	6
Wood[10]	Solitary	17
	Localized	11
	Extensive	3
Pettavel[11]	Solitary	22
	Few	11
	Numerous	5
	Extensive	1
Nielsen[12]	Few	18
	Several	9
	Numerous	5

* represent mean survival except for those of Kemeny et al, which is median survival.

is assessed by a surgeon during exploratory laparotomy. If there is a disagreement between preoperative and surgical assessment of the extent of liver involvement, the patient is rerandomized.

All patients undergo exploratory laparatomy not only for the placement of a hepatic artery catheter and Infusaid pump but also to ensure that two arms of the study are comparable by accurately defining the extent of liver involvement and assuring that there is no disease outside the liver. Any patient with a resectable hepatic lesion or extrahepatic disease is considered ineligible for the protocol. Many patients are now referred to the institution requesting the implantable pump. Consequently, not offering all patients the opportunity to receive a pump would greatly impair the accrual to the study.

Patients randomized to the intrahepatic therapy have the hepatic artery catheter connected to the pump. In the systemic group, the hepatic catheter is connected to an infus-a-port, and the pump is connected to an additional catheter placed in the cephalic vein (Fig. 1). If the disease progressed in a patient

Figure 1. Placement of Catheter and Infusaid Pump.

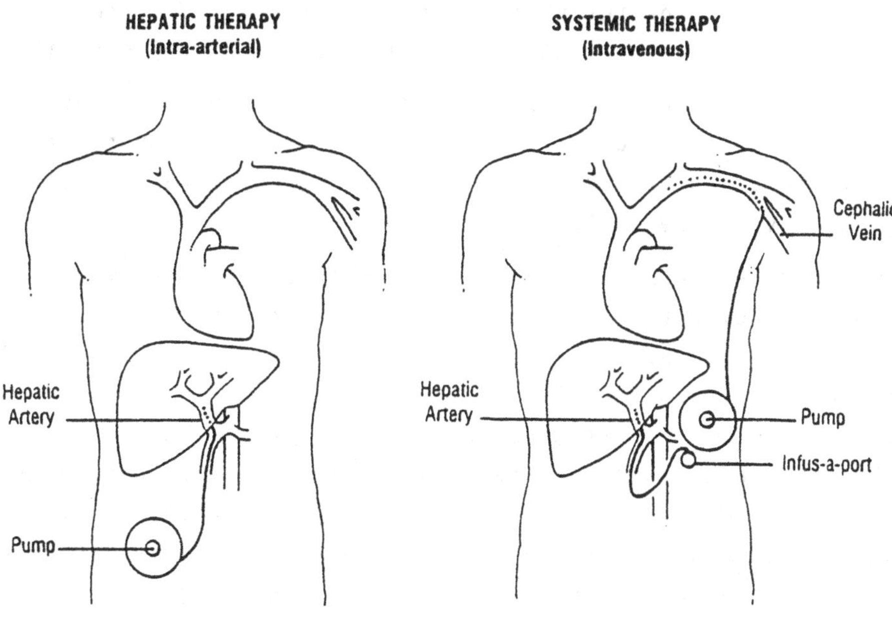

Figure 2. Conversion of Systemic to Hepatic Infusion Therapy.

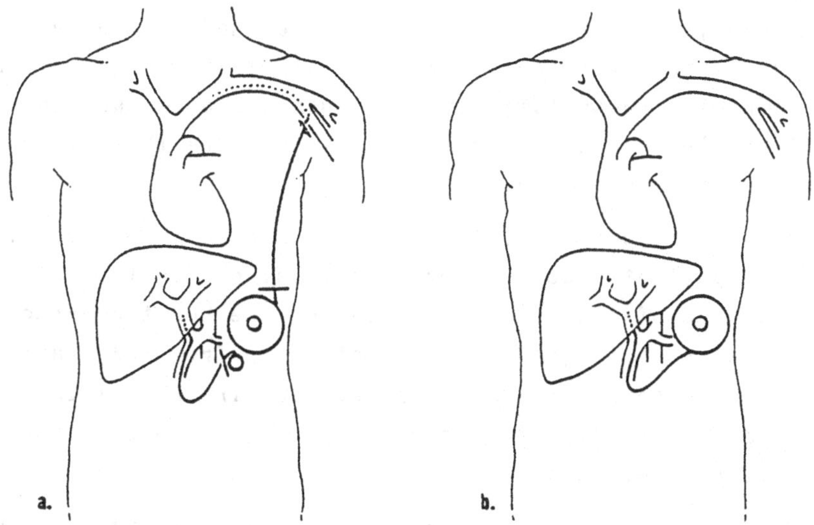

Patients whose disease progress on systemic infusion will have the pump catheter cut at 6 cm from the pump and spliced to the intrahepatic catheter.

in the latter group, a minor surgical procedure would allow a cross-over to the intrahepatic therapy (Fig. 2), thereby also allowing further evaluation of the efficacy of regional therapy.

The drug, FUDR, is administered by continuous infusion for 14 days via an infusaid pump in both groups. However, the starting doses is 0.30 mg/Kg/day for intrahepatic and 0.15 mg/Kg/day for systemic infusion.

Sixty-five patients have been referred for entry into the study. Four patients refused randomization, and 3 were excluded because of anomalous arterial blood supply, i.e. more than 3 vessels perfused the liver. Therefore, 58 patients were randomized preoperatively. Sixteen patients were excluded from the study after surgical exploration for the following reasons; resectable disease in 8 patients, extrahepatic disease in 7, and intra-abdominal infection in 1. Forty-two patients, therefore, have had the pump placed in the randomized study. The two groups were comparable (Table 3); they were well matched with respect to the percent liver involvement, initial laboratory values, PS, age and unfavorable prognostic factors (Table 4). Sex was the only parameter by which they were not well matched; there were only 2 females in the intrahepatic group, while 11/23 (48%) patients were women in the systemic group. When the data was analyzed to see if sex influenced the response, it appears that sex does not affect the response rate.

At the present time, 14 patients in each group are evaluable ble. Two patients had inadequate trials; one in the intrahepatic group because of incorrect placement of the hepatic catheter, and one in the systemic group because of death from very rapidly progressing disease in 3 weeks after starting FUDR infusion. The remaining 12 patients (4 in the intrahepatic and 8 in the systemic) are too early to evaluate.

Responses are assessed in the following manner. A complete response denotes the disappearance of all evidence of disease by CTT, liver scan, physical examination, blood chemistry profile, and CEA level. A partial response (PR) is defined as a greater

Table 3. Comparison of Patient Characteristics in Two Groups.

Characteristics	Intrahepatic (N=19)	Systemic (N=23)
Age (years)	62*	62
% Female	11%	48%
Karnofsky PS (%)	80	80
Initial laboratory data		
Alk. phosphatase (U/l)	213	213
LDH (U/l)	398	449
CEA (ng/ml)	73	178
Albumin (gm/dl)	4.0	4.1

* all numbers represent medians except % female

Table 4. Comparison of Unfavorable Patient Characterisctics in Two Groups.

Unfavorable Characteristics		Intrahepatic (N=19)	Systemic (N=23)
Palpable liver		11	12
Liver involvement	≥50%	8	12
Karnofsky PS	≤70%	4	3
Initial laboratory data			
LDH	≥500 U/l	6	10
CEA	≥100 ng/ml	9	13
WBC	≥10,000 cells/mm^3	3	4
Albumin	<4.0 gm/dl	8	7
Alk. phos.	≥300 U/l	5	5

than 50% reduction in the size of measurable disease by CTT or liver scan. If the liver is palpable, a 50% reduction in liver measurements is also required. A minor response (MR) is a 25-50% reduction in the size of measurable disease. CEA reductions are noted but are not used to define a response.

There have been 6 PRs in 14 evaluable patients in the intrahepatic group and 5 PRs in 14 evaluable patients in the systemic group. The median duration of response is 6 months for the intrahepatic group and 5 months for the systemic group. There is one MR in each group. In the systemic group, 2 patients

Table 5. Comparison of Therapeutic Response in Two Groups.

	Intrahepatic	Systemic
TOTAL ENTERED	19	23
Too early to evaluate	4	8
Inadequate trial	1	1
EVALUABLE	14	14
Partial Response	6	5
Minor Response	1	1
Stable	0	2 (3+, 12+)
CEA reduction >50%	8	6

* duration of response in months

have stable disease for 12+ and 3+ months. Eight of 16 patients in the intrahepatic group and 6/17 patients in the systemic grou have had more than 50% reduction in CEA level (Table 5).

Five patients who had failed to respond to the systemic treatment have been crossed-over to the intrahepatic treatment. One patient had a very transient improvement in liver function tests, which was followed by thrombosis of the hepatic artery an progression of disease. Three patients have failed to respond t intrahepatic infusion of FUDR after cross-over and have received Mitomycin C via a sideport of the pump; one of them responded.

Although the starting dose for the intrahepatic therapy was twice as high as the systemic therapy, doses in both arms were quite similar after the third cycle of treatment. Five patients required a reduction in their doses after the first cycle of intrahepatic infusion, 6 after the second, and 4 after the third so the median dose after the third treatment was 0.20 mg/Kg/day for 14 days. In the systemic arm, the starting dose was 0.15 mg/Kg/day x 14 days in the first 9 patients. Five of these patients developed diarrhea (severe in 2), which required a reduction of dose to 0.125 mg/Kg/day x 14 days. Then, subsequen patients were started on a dose of 0.125 mg/Kg/day x 14 days. Among 14 patients started on this dose, 7 have already tolerated an increased dose of 0.15 mg/Kg/day x 14 days, and 3 have not received their second dose. Therefore, the median dose at the present time for the systemic group is 0.15 mg/Kg/day x 14 days.

Table 6. Comparison of Toxicity in Two Groups.

Toxicity	Intrahepatic (N=14*)	Systemic (N=14*)
Ulcer	4	0
Diffuse gastritis	1	0
SGOT elevation, >100%	7	0
Bilirubin elevation, >3.0 mg/dl	2	0
Diarrhea	0	9
Colitis	0	2

* evaluable patients

The toxicity has been quite different between the 2 groups (Table 6). In the intrahepatic group, the toxicity has been mainly gastro-intestinal and hepatic. Four (29%) of 14 patients developed significant gastrointestinal ulcers documented by endoscopy, and a fifth patient had severe gastritis. Seven (50%) patients developed an elevation of SGOT greater than 100% over baseline value, and two developed a significant elevation of serum bilirubin (9.0 and 10.0 mg/dl, respectively). In the systemic group, the major toxicity has been diarrhea - seen in 9/14 (64%) adequately treated patients. In 2 patients, sigmoidoscopy revealed sigmoid ulcerations suggestive of colitis. Both patients required hospitalization for supportive care including IV hydration.

Another significant difference between the 2 groups was the development of extrahepatic disease. In the intrahepatic group, 10 patients have already developed extrahepatic disease (6 lung, 3 intraabdominal and 1 bone). At the present time, no patients in the systemic group have developed extrahepatic disease.

There has been no difference in survival between the 2 treatment groups. However, this study is still in the early phase; only 5 patients in the intrahepatic group and 3 in the systemic group have died. The median survival, at the present time, for the intrahepatic group is 11 months, while it has not been reached for the systemic group because of limited follow-up thus far and very few deaths.

CONCLUSIONS

Although it is still too early to reach definite conclusions, the following observations on the infusional chemotherapy in hepatic metastases from colorectal carcinoma can be made:

1) The response rates for the intrahepatic and systemic infusions are similar.
2) The development of extrahepatic disease is common with intrahepatic infusion and thus far has not been observed in the systemic infusion group.
3) Gastrointestinal toxicity is common with both types of infusion; upper gastrointestinal ulceration is observed with intrahepatic infusion, whereas diarrhea is observed with systemic infusion.

REFERENCES

1. Kemeny N, Yagoda A, Braun D, Golbey R: Therapy for metastatic colorectal carcinoma with a combination of Methyl-CCNU, 5-Fluorouracil, Vincristine, and Streptozotocin (MOF-Strep). Cancer (45): 876-881, 1980.
2. Bengmark S, Hafstrom L: The natural history of primary and secondary malignant tumors of the liver. Cancer (23): 198-202, 1969.
3. Kemeny N: The systemic chemotherapy of hepatic metastases. Sem Oncol (10): 148-158, 1983.
4. Breedis C, Young G: The blood supply of neoplasms in the liver. Am J Path (30): 969-985, 1954.
5. Ensminger W, Rosowsky A, Raso V, Levin D, Glode M, Come S, Steele G, Frei E: A clinical-pharmacological evaluation of hepatic arterial infusions of 5-fluoro-2'-deoxyuridine and 5-fluorouracil. Cancer Res (38): 3784-3792, 1978.
6. Ensminger W, Niederhuber J, Gyves J, Thrall J, Cozzi E, Doan K: Effective control of liver metastases from colon cancer with an implanted system for hepatic arterial chemotherapy. Proc ASCO (1): 94, 1982.
7. Kemeny N, Daly J, Oderman P, Shike M, Chun H, Petroni G, Geller N: Hepatic artery pump infusion: Toxicity and results in patients with metastatic colorectal carcinoma. J Clin Oncol (In press).
8. Cady B, Oberfield RA: Regional infusion chemotherapy of hepatic metastases from carcinoma of the colon. Am J Surg (127): 220-227, 1974.

9. Kemeny N, Braun DW: Prognostic factors in advanced colorectal carcinoma. Importance of lactic dehydrogenage, performance status and white blood cell count. Am J Med (74): 786-797, 1983.
10. Wood CB, Gillis CR, Blumgart LH: A retrospective study of the natural history of patients with liver metastases from colorectal cancer. Clin Oncol (2): 285-288, 1976.
11. Pettavel J, Morgenthaler F: Protracted arterial chemotherapy of liver tumors: An experience of 107 cases over a 12-year period. In: Ariel IM (ed) Progress in Clinical Cancer. Grune & Stratton, New York, 1978, pp 217-233.
12. Nielsen J, Balslev I, Jensen HE: Carcinoma of the colon with liver metastases. Acta Chir Scand (137): 463-465, 1971.

THE RATIONALE AND METHODOLOGY FOR INTRA-ARTERIAL CHEMOTHERAPY WITH BCNU AS TREATMENT FOR GLIOBLASTOMA

Fred H. Hochberg, M.D.; Amy Pruitt, M.D. Deborah Beck, M.D.;G. DeBruyn, M.D.; Kenneth Davis, M.D.
From the Services of Neurology (FH,AP,DB) and Radiology (GDB, KD), Massachusetts General Hospital. Supported by the Naragansett Foundation and the Farber and Sanford Funds.

ABSTRACT

The rationale, methodology and early experience with intra-arterial infusion of BCNU will be described. Internal carotid artery BCNU is now used as standard therapy for post-operative glioblastoma in at least five institutions. The approach allows for five-fold multiples of drug into localized intracerebral tumor without increasing systemic toxicity. Major complications are limited to ipsilateral eye pain and diminished acuity treated with systemic analgesia, retro-orbital bipuvacaine block or avoided by supra-ophthalmic carotid artery infusion. However, the latter is associated with leukoencephalopathic changes seen as low absorption on CT scan. We will present our experience with 171 infusions of BCNU amongst 54 patients including:

a) Patients with post-operative and post-irradiation recurrent glioblastoma who experienced 54 weeks median survival following recurrence.
b) Patients with newly diagnosed and irradiated glioblastoma who have median survival of 53+ weeks(following infraopthalmic infusion) and 56+ weeks (for three or more supraophthalmic artery infusions)
c) Patients receiving intra-arterial BCNU in advance of irradiation.

Intra-arterial BCNU represents a safe and easily performed technique for treatment of glioblastoma. Despite twenty-two years of clinical use, BCNU has been shown to be no more than marginally effective in the treatment of glioblastoma. In controlled studies (14), BCNU administered by vein at doses of 240mg/m^2 is associated with only 20% improvement in length of survival when added to irradiation in patients who have had tumor biopsy or resection. No clear evidence of improvement in quality of life has been noted (6). These data stand in contrast to qualities that make BCNU a theoretically ideal drug for the treatment of intracranial tumors: its high lipid solubility and short half life, its steep dose — response relationship in tissue culture and animal systems in which glial tumors are targets, and its effectiveness against intracranial tumors in animal studies. Major dose limitations exist for BCNU (10). Cumulative and single doses in excess of 1500mg/m^2 have been associated with toxicities involving kidney (50% of patients), lung (20%), liver (10%) and central nervous system (2%). These complications are in addition to characteristic dose-related and cumulative myelo-suppression. The resulting leukopenia and thrombocytopenia are noted with single intravenous doses of BCNU in excess of 400mg/m^2 and are severe above 600mg/m^2.

Attempts to circumvent this myelo-suppression have involved the infusion of frozen or refrigerated autologous bone marrow harvested prior to high dose BCNU chemotherapy (3,5). Although allowing BCNU administration at single dose levels in excess of 1400mg/m^2, these approaches are cumbersome and associated with significant non-marrow toxicity.

The Rationale for Intra-arterial Therapy with BCNU

Four facts provide the rationale for arterial infusion of

BCNU in the treatment of glioblastoma:

1. Regional therapy is a logical approach to therapy of a "regional disease." Glioblastoma (with the exception of the 4% which are multicentric) is a "localized" malignancy often well defined by computed tomographic techniques (4). Arteriography can identify feeding arteries which are most often within the distribution of the internal carotid artery. Exceptions are malignant pontine tumors or the rare (12), subarachnoid or systemic metastases of glioblastoma in children.

2. The major dose limitations to BCNU administration result from non-central nervous system toxicities(7). Arterial administration of BCNU allows for higher regional drug levels without increasing the risk of systemic toxicity.

3. BCNU represents an excellent drug choice for regional arterial infusion by virtue of a short half life, lipid solubility and steep dose response relationship in model systems of brain malignancies.

4. Familiar, well established angiographic techniques allow for easy, rapid and low morbidity drug infusions. These safe techniques now include those involving catheterization of the supra-ophthalimic carotid artery.

These facts led investigators to explore intra-arterial administration of BCNU in experimental models. Levin (9) and associates, using ^{14}C labeled BCNU, demonstrated brain concentrations of BCNU four times greater following arterial (carotid) infusion than following intravenous administration and Fenstermacher (1) predicted that brain levels might be as high as ten-fold greater without increased bone marrow exposure. The availability of high-performance liquid chromatography assays for BCNU (8) have confirmed these studies.

The Arterial Administration of BCNU

West and Madajewicz(11,15), in 1979, began to use

intra-arterial infusions of BCNU and other agents to treat both glioblastoma and central nervous system metastases. Their experience with over 150 infusions, usually intra-carotid, provided the impetus for workers at the University of Michigan (2) and at the Massachusetts General Hospital to study intra-arterial therapy of glioblastoma in patients with newly diagnosed and recurrent tumors.

At the Massachusetts General Hospital, arterial BCNU therapy has been used to treat 54 patients in 171 infusions. Our initial experience with the treatment of 12 patients with recurrent glioblastoma after surgery and radiation therapy provided a 54+ week survival from recurrence and 94 weeks from the date of diagnosis. Our current approach involves the treatment of patients with biopsy-proven glioblastoma who have not yet had irradiation. Patients are included in the protocol if:

A. There is no evidence of bleeding within the tumor as assessed by CT scan.
B. There is no arterial contraindiction to infusion (carotid stenosis, carotid dissection) or to BCNU therapy [prior chemotherapy, bleeding diathesis, leukopenia, (WBC<3000), thrombocytopenia (platelets<150,000)].
C. The tumor has shown no evidence of subarachnoid dissemination by CT scan.(Tumor within the territory of more than one intracranial artery is a relative contraindication)
D. Karnofsky status is greater than 70% at outset.
E. Progression of cerebral edema necessitating increased steroid doses has not been noted two weeks prior to infusion.

PREVIOUS EXPERIENCE WITH INTRA-ARTERIAL BCNU
Protocol I (Recurrent glioblastoma - infraophthalmic arterial)

Patients: Recurrent glioblastoma (post-operative, post-irradiation >5 months)

Drug Dose: Dose escalation BCNU ($250mg/m^2$, $350mg/m^2$, 450mg/m2, 600mg/m2). Three patients at each dose level.

Dose Frequency: Every 5-6 weeks

Administration technique: Infraophthalmic carotid infusion

Protocal II (Newly diagnosed glioblastoma infraophthalmic versus supraophthalmic carotid)

Patients: Newly diagnosed glioblastoma (post-operative, post-irradiation)

Drug Dose: BCNU $240mg/m^2$

Dose Frequency: Every 5-6 weeks

Administration: Supraophthalmic carotid via DeBruyn balloon

Protocol III (Newly Diagnosed Glioblastoma Prior to Irradiation)

Patients:Biopsy-proven glioblastoma

Drug Dose: 240mg/m2

Dose Frequency:Every 4 weeks for 4 infusions. Followed by Irradiation. Provision for irradiation if chemotherapy failure before week 16.

Administration: Either infra-or supraophthalmic infusion as above

For all infusions, on the morning of chemotherapy an intravenous line is inserted, and the patient is not fed. Premedication is 5mg of intramuscular morphine sulfate. Infusion makes use of a Seldinger technique percutaneous transfemoral retrograde catheterization of the internal carotid artery at the level of C2 or the supra-ophthalmic carotid artery often to the bifurcation of the middle cerebral artery. This latter catheterization makes use of the DeBruyn calibrated leak balloon. A silastic catheter (of 0.4mm internal and 0.8mm external diameters), ending in the fenestrated balloon, passes within a 7F polyethylene introducer (Ingenor, 70 Rue Orfila, 75020 Paris, France). The balloon does not inflate during the infusion of BCNU and never occludes the vessel during the procedure, which is performed under systemic heparinization. The neurologist present during the procedure mixes the BCNU (100mgs of BCNU/1cc of alcohol) and dilutes it into 125 ccs of normal saline. The mixture is continuously agitated in the darkened room and is pump infused at 2 to 3 ccs/minute. Post infusion nausea is treated with intramuscular Compazine. Infusion-related brain swelling is treated by the post-infusion intravenous administration of Solumedrol (80 mg). Infra-ophthalmic infusions are associated with eye pain, conjunctival injection, erythema and unilateral rhinorrhea in patients. This retro-orbital pain may be diminished by reduction of the alcohol content (which may reduce the amount of drug in solution), the substituion of DMSO solvent, the addition of intravenous morphine sulfate (to 15 mg) or the use of a retro-orbital block using a one-to-one mixture of 0.5 percent bipuvacaine and two percent xylocaine with epinephrine administered by an ophthalmologist (Dr. Kambiz Moused, M.D. unpublished data). In all instances, eye pain resolved within 10 minutes of the end of infusion, but one patient experienced diminished visual acuity to 29/40 in the eye, and retinal infarction was seen. A second patient with pre-existing bilateral papilledema experienced bilateral loss of vision with a similar fundoscopic picture. The supra-ophthalmic infusions are associated with lateral head pain in 10 percent of patients and a somewhat higher frequency of seizure activity (Table 1). CT scan low-absorption changes surrounding the tumor site are noted within 2 weeks of infusion and may represent specific drug-related leukoencephalopathy in the previously irradiated patients.

TABLE 1
COMPLICATIONS OF BCNU INFUSION

	Infra-ophthalmic	Supra-ophthalmic
Patients	36	18
Infusions	113	31
Eye Pain	113	10% (Lateral head)
Seizures	2	2
Blindness	1	0
Retinal Change	3	0
Tumor Hemorrhage	2	0
Low Absorption (Edema/Leukoencephalopathy)	0	7
Spread Out of Arterial Site	0	2
Stroke (MCA)	0	2
Hematologic Toxicity	0	0
Miscellaneous	Carotid Dissection	

Surprisingly, BCNU associated leukopenia, pulmonary toxicity and hepatic toxicity have not been significant. Cumulative doses of BCNU have been kept below 1,250 mgs of BCNU/meters^2.

RESULTS

One hundred seventy one infusions (113 infra-ophthalmic and 58 supra-ophthalmic) have been performed on 55 patients. We are currently performing 3 to 5 infusions per week.

Protocol 1. (Recurrent glioblastoma)(13). Twelve patients received 37 infusions of BCNU through an infra-ophthalmic route as part of this protocol. There was no significant difference in immediate toxicity between dose levels, and doses to 600 mg/meter^2 could successfully be infused. This patient population has been followed through 164 weeks (as of Jan 1984). The median survival for the population following recurrence is 54 weeks. Eleven of the twelve patients were alive one year from the date of their recurrence, and three are still alive almost three years from their tumor recurrence. These three continue to show contrast-enhancing abnormalities of smaller size than noticed previously.

Protocol II. Infraophthalmic Infusions: We have treated twenty-four patients through 76 infusions of BCNU into infra-ophthalmic carotid sites for newly diagnosed and irradiated glioblastoma. These patients have been followed for 124 weeks (through 1/84). The median survival is 48+ weeks. Of the patients completing 3 or more infusions, median survival is 53+ weeks. The longest survivors are now 127+, 123+, 121+, 119+, 119+ . No patient removed himself from the protocol. Patients removed because of tratment-related complications included one patient with asthma and one with a small hemorrhage into his tumor. Although patients succumbed to non-treatment-related pulmonary embolus and infection (one patient each), nine of the patients have developed recurrent tumor within the original vascular distribution.

Supraophthalmic Infusions: We have treated eighteen patients through 58 infusions following diagnosis and irradiation. These infusions have involved placement of balloon-guided catheters into the supraophthalmic carotid, often as far as the first division of the middle cerebral artery. Followed through Jan 1984, this group has a median survival of 41+ weeks. Twelve patients received more than 3 infusions. The median survival for this subgroup is 56+ weeks. The longest survivors for this sub group are alive 127+, 119+, and 102+ weeks from the date of diagnosis.

Protocol III: We have entered two patients through three infusions. We expect no increased toxicity in this population, providing that sufficient time has elapsed to provide post-surgical recovery.

DISCUSSION

At a time when pessimism continues to surround the therapy of malignant glioma, the introduction of intra-arterial chemotherapy allows BCNU concentrations fivefold greater than those following intravenous administratin. Our initial experience demonstrates the feasibility of infra-ophthalmic carotid infusion of BCNU to 600 mgs/meters^2. Concerns regarding ophthalmic toxicity, however, caused three of us (FH,GdeB,KD) to seek supra-ophthalmic infusion techniques (16,17). The availability of a balloon guidance system has enabled us to perform these supra-ophthalmic and selective middle and anterior cerebral artery infusions in excess of 50 times. This infusion technique avoids both immediate eye pain and ophthalmic toxicity. It carries with it, however, the risk of worsened cerebral edema and the possible association of leukoencephalopathy in previously irradiated patients. It is for this reason that Protocol 3 (pre-irradiation) was constructed, thereby avoiding the effects of prior irradiation:hyalinized blood vessels, increased cerebral edema, foci of necrosis within tumor tissue.

This approach provides the patient with BCNU 240mg/m2 every four weeks, beginning 3 weeks after craniotomy but prior to irradiation. With four administrations of drug (either by infra-or supraophthalmic infusion) we are able to provide 960 mg BCNU/m2 in the 19 weeks following operation. Thus irradiation is delayed for slightly over 4 months at a time when patient quality of life is expected to be maximized. (This approach avoids the institution of 35 daily doses of irradiation to patients who have already been hospitalized for craniotomy and post-operative care.) Standard field and dose irradiation is provided following the fourth infusion OR IN THE EVENT of CT or clinical deterioration prior to that time. This approach, involving low systemic doses of BCNU, thereby avoids hematologic, pulmonary, and renal complications associated with cumulative doses of the drug above 1250 mg/m2. It involves only 1.5 days of hospitalization for the 2 hour infusion procedure.

REFERENCES

1. Fenstermacher, JD, Cowless, AL: Theoretic Limitation of Intracarotid Infusions in Brain Tumor Chemotherapy. Cancer Treat Rep 61: 519-526, 1977.

2. Greenberg, HS, Ensiminger, WD, Seeger, JF, et al: Intra-arterial BCNU Chemotherapy for the Treatment of Malignant Gliomas of the Central Nervous System: A preliminary report. Cancer Treat Rep 65: 803-810, 1981.

3. Herzig, GP, Phillips, GL, Herzig, RH, et al: High-dose Nitrosourea (BCNU) and Autologous Bone Marrow Transplantation: A Phase I Study _in_ Nitrosoureas: Current Status and New Developments, Prestayko, AW, Crooke, ST, Baker, LH, et al. (eds.), New York Academic Press, pp 337-341, 1981.

4. Hochberg, FH, and Pruitt, A: Assumptions in the Radiotherapy of Glioblastoma: Neurology 30: 901-911, 1980.

5. Hochberg, FH, Parker, LM, Takvorian, T., et al.: High-dose BCNU with Autologous bone marrow rescue for recurrent glioblastoma multiforme. J Neurosurg 54: 455-460, 1981.

6. Hochberg, FH, Linggood, R, Wolfson, L, et al.: Quality and Duration of Survival in Glioblastoma Multiforme. Combined Surgical, Radiation, and Lomustine Therapy. JAMA 241: 1016-1018, 1979.

7. Kapp, J, Vance, R, Parker, JL, and Smith, RR: Complications of High-dose Intra-arterial BCNU Chemotherapy for Malignant Glioma. Congress of neurological Surgeons, Neurosurg 9: 472-473, 1981 (abstr).

8. Krull, IS, Strauss, J, Hochberg, FH, et al.: An Improved Trace Analysis for N-Nitrosoureas from Biological Media. Analyt Toxicol 5: 42=46, 1981.

9. Levin, VA, Kabra, PM, Freeman-Dove, MA: Pharmacokinetics of Intra-carotid Arter C^{14} -BCNU in the squirrel monkey. J Neurosurg 48: 587, 1978.

10. MacDonald, JS, Weiss, RB, Poster, D, et al: Subacute and Chronic Toxicities Associated with Nitrosourea Therapy in Nitrosoureas: Current Status and New Developments, Prestayko, AW, Crooke, ST, Baker, LH, et al. (eds.), New York Academic Press, pp 145-154, 1981.

11. Madajewicz, S, West, CR, Park, HC, et al.: Phase II study - Intra-arterial BCNU Therapy for Metastic Brain Tumors. Cancer 47: 653-657, 1980.

12. Pasquier, B, Pasquier, D, N'Golet, A, et al.: Extraneural Metastases of Astrocytomas and Glioblastomas: Clinicopathological Study of Two Cases and Review of Literature. Cancer 45: 112-125, 1980.

13. Pruitt, A, Hochberg, FH, Grossman, R, Davis, K: Intracarotid BCNU Therapy for Recurrent Glioblastomas: A Phase II Dose Escalation Study in 12 Patients With Recurrent Glioblastoma. Presented at TOTALLY IMPLANTABLE DRUG DELIVERY SYSTEM CONFERENCE, Saddlebrook, Florida, March, 1983 (Infusaid Corporation and University of Michigan Medical Center, Ann Arbor, Mich)

14. Walker, D, Green, SB, Byar, DP, et al.: Randomized Comparisons of Radiotherapy and Nitrosoureas for the Treatment of Malignant Glioma After Surgery. N Eng J Med 303: 1323-1329, 1980.

15. West, CR, Yamada, K, Karakousis, CP, et al.: Intra-arterial BCNU Infusion for Intracerebral Metastases from Malignant Melanoma and Lung Cancer. Proc Am Accoc Cancer Res and ASCO 20: 332, 1979.

16. DeBrun, G.M., Vinuela, FV, Foc, AJ and Kan, S: Two Different Calibrated Leak Balloons. Amer. Jnl. Neuroradiology 3: 407-414, 1982.

17. DeBrun, GM, Davis, KR and Hochberg, FH: Amer Jnl. Neuroradiology, May-June, 1983, in press.

INTRA-ARTERIAL CIS-PLATINUM IN ADVANCED SOLID TUMORS

DANIEL E. LEHANE, M.D.

INTRODUCTION

Since cis-platinum was introduced as a chemotherapeutic agent, there have been many pharmacologic manipulations utilized to improve its therapeutic index. Initially, efforts were directed toward reducing toxicity. Dose-limiting nephrotoxicity has been successfully ameliorated by a variety of hydration schema including mannitol diuresis, sodium thiosulfate administration and the use of hypertonic saline.[1,2,3] Severe nausea and vomiting have been avoided using metoclopramide and other anti-emitics.[4] Second generation anologues with less nephrotoxicity are now being studied.[5] These efforts have succeeded in improving the therapeutic index for cis-platinum to some degree by reducing toxicity and thereby increasing the maximum tolerated dose.

In 1979 the effectiveness of intra-arterial cis-platinum (IACP) administration in patients with advanced malignancies was reported. Subsequently it has been demonstrated that the intra-arterial administration of cis-platinum is associated with increased response rates ranging from 2-to 10-fold over intravenous administration of the drug in the same diseases. The effective uses of IACP have been documented in patients with melanomas, soft tissue sarcomas, squamous cell carcinomas of the head and neck region, gynecologic tumors, carcinomas of the colon, primary malignant gliomas, adenoidcystic carcinoma, carcinoma of the prostate, bladder carcinoma, and perhaps carcinoma of the breast, lung and hepatoma.[6,7,8,9,10,11,12,13,14,15,16,17] The initial clinical series using IACP reported an increased response rate in patients with advanced, regional melanoma.[7] Anticipated results for intravenous cis-platinum administration range from 10 to 25% in patients with malignant melanoma, and the results using IACP were shown to be approximately 50%. Later reports described a high response rate of approximately 50% in patients with soft tissue and bony sarcomas, permitting limb salvage surgery and providing dramatic pain relief in many patients.[8] These results emphasized the marked increase in therapeutic activity of cis-platinum when given by intra-arterial infusion. This paper will describe these and other clinical series where the effectiveness of IACP administration is demonstrated. These results suggest that an improved therapeutic index for cis-platinum may be achieved by increasing the therapeutic activity

Methods

All patients had histologically confirmed malignancy which was not amenable to alternate forms of therapy and gave their informed consent to receive such treatment. IACP was infused via intra-arterial catheters placed using the Seldinger technique, and all catheters were removed following treatment. Catheters were replaced for second and third infusions using the same technique.

In an effort to avoid nephrotoxicity, a simple hydration scheme was utilized. Mannitol diuresis was not routinely employed. However, patients with large brain tumors were given mannitol, 12.5 grams intravenously every 4 to 6 hours beginning 2 hours after cis-platinum infusion in an effort to control anticipated cerebral edema in these patients. Prehydration was accomplished using 0.2% NaCl given at 200cc/hr for 3 to 12 hours pre-infusion and usually resulted in a water diuresis. Following cis-platinum administration, hydration was continued intravenously for 24 to 48 hours using 0.2% NaCl until patients were able to maintain an oral hydration rate of 3 liters per 24 hours, which was then continued for 1 week. Cis-platinum was prepared as a 1mg/ml solution using 0.9% NaCl as diluent. Cis-platinum solutions were prepared immediately prior to infusion and were filtered using a 0.2

micron filter prior to its use. Cis-platinum was administered at a dose of $100mg/m^2$ for patients with a creatinine clearance of 70cc/min or greater. Patients with a creatinine clearance of 45 to 70cc/min had a dose reduction calculated as follows: dose = Ccr in cc-min x BSA in m^2, ie., for patients with creatinine clearance of 50cc/min, cis-platinum was given at a dose of $50mg/m^2$. Appropriate reductions in cis-platinum dose were made for second and third infusions in responding patients if their creatinine clearances fell during treatment. Cis-platinum was repeated at 4-week intervals. While other investigators have used cis-platinum infusion rates ranging from 1 to 4 hours, and even as long as 24 hours in an effort to ameliorate nausea, we have used a 1 -hour infusion time for all patients. Anti-emetics were used liberally prior to and during infusion, and the use of metoclopramide, 3mg/kg immediately prior to cis-platinum infusion and repeated at 2 hours, has made a dramatic impact on reducing nausea to a very acceptable level. Nephrotoxins, such as aminoglycoside antibiotics and diuretics, are avoided when possible.

We feel that filtration of the drug has significantly lowered the incidence of CNS toxicity, but we have recognized that patients with large CNS mass lesions who receive IACP frequently experience a large amount of cerebral edema in and surrounding the tumor mass, which may produce significant symptoms.[12] We have been able to successfully control this rebound cerebral edema using mannitol following cis-platinum infusion for patients in whom this is anticipated. All patients who received CNS infusions received prophylactic dexamethasone (5 to $10mg/m^2$) twice daily and anti-convulsant therapy. Vertebral artery infusion is associated with complete, unresolving deafness and is thus contra-indicated. Patients with tumors in the head and neck region may also experience sudden edema, which may result in cranial nerve palsies, especially as a result of parotid gland swelling. In an effort to avoid this problem, many patients also receive prophylactic dexamethasone pre-treatment. Patients with head and neck tumors may receive selective arterial infusions or regional redistribution of blood flow using non-detachable baloon catheters or gelfoam embolae in an effort to concentrate the arterial infusion in the tumor-bearing area. In other locations throughout the body, either multiple, selective vessel infusions or embolae-produced redistribution of blood flow is employed when necessary.

Results

Melanoma: The initial series reported by Prichard et al. (4 patients) and Calvo et al. (19 patients) described a total of 23 patients with recurrent melanoma, all but 4 of whom had received prior chemotherapy.[6,7] They described an overall response rate of 52% (2/4 and 10/19), including 4 patients who achieved a complete response. In our own series we have treated an additional 13 patients with regionally confined melanoma, with 6 responses. Two of these patients have achieved a complete response; 1 with liver metastases, who continued in complete loco-regional response confirmed at autopsy, and 1 with axillary metastases.

Sarcomas: Initially Calvo et al. reported 10 patients and later Mavligit et al. 23 patients with inoperable predominately skeletal sarcomas and found a 52% response rate using IACP.[6,8] They reported the use of pre-operative infusions that permitted salvage surgery and a dramatic relief of pain in some patients. In our own series, we have treated 14 patients with advanced sarcomas, with 8 responses, including 6 patients with malignant fibrous histiocytoma, 3 of whom responded.

TABLE 1 OVERALL EXPERIENCE
BAYLOR COLLEGE OF MEDICINE
INTRA-ARTERIAL CIS-PLATINUM 1-1-84

PRIMARY SITE	#RX	#Resp	%
H&N	68	64	94%
Colon	65	43**	75%
Lung	16	9	56%
Melanoma	13	6	46%
Sq Skin	3	3	-
Sarcoma	8	5	63%
Fibrous Histiocytoma	6	3	50%
Adenoidcystic	3	2	67%
Bladder	3	1	-
Prostate	2	2	-
Hepatoma	9	7	-
Testes	1	0	-
Sq Rectum	1	0	-
Glioblastoma	57	8***	67%
Pancreas	2	0	-
Breast	3	0	-
Salivary/mixed	1	1	-
Ovarian	1	1	-
Cervix	1	1	-
Lymphoma	2	1	-
Chordoma	2	1	-
Pinealoma	1	1	-
Total	264	159	

** = 8 adjuvant - not evaluable for response
*** = 38 adjuvant - not evaluable for response

Squamous-cell carcinoma of the head and neck region: We have reported a high response rate for patients with advanced squamous-cell carcinoma of the head and neck region using IACP.[9] Patients with head and neck cancer, who to date total 68, are divided into 3 groups based on stage and prior treatment. Of 26 patients with recurrent disease following prior treatment which included radiation therapy, 23 responded, with a median survival of 10 months. Of 34 patients with nonresectable Stage III and IV disease receiving IACP plus radiation therapy, 33 responded to chemotherapy, with a 14-month median survival. In this subgroup of patients, IACP was given 1 to 4 days prior to the start of radiotherapy, 4 weeks later at midpoint of radiotherapy and approximately 2 weeks after completing radiotherapy.

There was no evidence of additive mucous membrane toxicity or other unusual radiation cis-platinum toxicity noted in these patients. Patients in this subgroup who presented with nasopharyngeal carcinomas also received post-treatment methotrexate maintenance for 9 months following completion of cis-platinum. The subgroup of patients with nasopharyngeal carcinoma has experienced a prolonged survival with a plateau in the survival curve at 62%,which begins at 18 months after the start of treatment and extends to 4 years of observation.

TABLE 2 SQUAMOUS CELL CARCINOMA HEAD & NECK REGION - IACP

Recurrent Disease			Stages III-IV+XRT			Stage III+Surg.		
1° Site	Resp.	Surv.Wks.	1° Site	Resp.	Surv.	1°Site	Resp.	Surv.
Max	PR	19	BOT	PR	56	BOT	PR	15
Ethmoid	PR	19	NPC	CR	86	Hypo P	PR	74
Pyricorm	PR	39	Epi	PR	56	MAX	PR	60
Max	PR	58	Palate	PR	21	Eth	CR	65
FOM	PR	12	BOT	PR	32	Oro P	PR	44
Tonsil	CR	20	Tonsil	PR	36	Hypo P	PR	116+
Palate	NR	4	FOM	PR	28	FOM	PR	156+
Hypo P	PR	17	Oro P	PR	24	Epi	PR	17
FOM	CR	67	BOT	CR	56			
Larynx	CR	47	Palate	CR	56			
Larynx	PR	45	FOM	PR	128+			
Nose	CR	157+	FOM	PR	104+			
Hypo P	PR	30	BOT	PR	20			
NPC	CR	192+	NPC	CR	108+			
Oro P	NR	69	NPC	CR	64			
NPC	CR	172+	BOT	PR	22			
Max	PR	20	Hypo P	PR	35			
Hypo P	CR	48	NPC	PR	61			
Max	PR	17	NPC	PR	40			
Hypo P	PR	22	Max	CR	128+			
NPC	PR	35	Oro P	NR	30			
NPC	CR	100+	NPC	CR	104+			
NPC	CR	100+	NPC	CR	108+			
BOT	CR	53+	Max	CR	62+			
Max	PR	39	Eth	PR	24			
Hypo P	NR	204	Hypo P	PR	104			
			NPC	CR	35+			
			NPC	CR	21+			
			NPC	CR	17+			
			NPC	PR	8+			
			NPC	PR	22+			
			NPC	CR	82+			
			NPC	CR	100+			
			NPC	CR	100+			
Totals	23/26	39 wks.		33/34	56 wks		8/8	60 wks

From these observations, we have concluded that IACP results in a higher response rate for patients with head and neck cancers, that it can be safely added at full dose to full-dose radiation therapy, and that this modality should be considered as a remission-inducing program which has a relatively small impact on survival (50% greater than predicted). We conclude that a maintenance treatment program will be necessary following the remission induction with IACP to improve overall survival. A small group of patients (8) with advanced resectable disease received pre-operative IACP. All responded to the chemotherapy prior to surgery. Median survival in this group is 60 weeks. We have found that this approach to head and neck cancer does not produce a therapeutic advantage over initiating treatment with surgery.

Response rates in squamous-cell carcinoma of the head and neck region are from 2 to 4 times greater than that reported in the literature for intravenous cis-platinum administration in comparably staged patients, and survival for these patients responding to intravenous or IACP is approximately 1½ times longer than predicted from studies using other effective regimens in similarly staged patients.

<u>Colon cancer:</u> The results of IACP for advanced metastatic colon cancer have been especially encouraging.[12] We have reported a 75% overall response rate, originally in a group of 36 patients which has now been increased to a total of 54 patients. This represents approximately a 10-fold increase in response rate compared to that reported for intravenous cis-platinum.[18] Survival was significantly prolonged for responders, with a median survival of 10 months compared to less than 3 months for nonresponders (p 0.001). This is the anticipated survival for similarly staged patients reported in the literature.[19] As can be seen in Table 3, which describes the pre-treatment characteristics of these patients, this series is heavily loaded with seriously ill, advanced-disease patients, the majority of whom received hepatic artery infusions for liver metastases. Despite the advanced stage of recurrent disease, the response rate in

this group is remarkably high, and survival is significantly prolonged. We have only a preliminary experience (8 patients) using IACP as an adjuvant therapy in patients with Dukes C carcinoma of the colon. It is as yet not determined in which anatomical region to apply intra-arterial chemotherapy in these patients. It was noted that in 14 patients from our original series who responded to IACP for recurrent disease in the liver, and who also had measurable disease in a distant uninfused site, no patients responded in these distant sites. Based on these observations, it is conceivable that adjuvant treatment with IACP for Dukes C carcinoma of the colon may provide local control of disease in the infused region, as in adjuvant hepatic artery infusions, while metastatic disease may become evident at distant sites, perhaps unusual to the natural history of the disease.

TABLE 3 COLON CANCER - IACP

Performance Status	Resp.	NonResp.	Prior Treatment	Resp.	NonResp.	Liver Function	Resp.	NonResp.
0-1	7	1	yes	16	7	Abnormal	13	5
2	17	3	no	26	5	Normal	29	7
3-4	18	8						

Brain tumors: The results of IACP in patients with malignant primary brain tumors are remarkable in view of the small amount of drug reported to cross the blood brain barrier. We have treated 38 patients with Grade III and IV malignant gliomas using an adjuvant post-operative IACP program. Preliminary analysis of this group of patients reveals a median survival of approximately 90 weeks, representing a more than 2-fold improvement in survival compared to that reported in the literature for similarly staged patients.[20] Approximately 40% of the patients treated in the first year of this series (2 of 5) remain free of disease after 3 years, and nearly 50% are alive after 2 years. In addition, 15 patients with recurrent, previously treated malignant gliomas received IACP, with a resulting 67% response rate and a median survival of 6 months, further confirming the therapeutic activity of IACP in primary brain tumors.

TABLE 4 IACP

ADJUVANT MALIGNANT GLIOMAS: PRETREATMENT CHARACTERISTICS

Age	#pts.	Sex	#pts.	Histologic Tumor Grade	#pts.
0-30	7	M	25	III	19
30-50	19	F	13	IV	16
50+	12				
Median 42					

Other tumor types: The data for patients with other types of cancer are less well developed. Carlson et al. reported 3/9 patients with advanced recurrent squamous-cell carcinomas of the uterine cervix, of whom 3 responded.(10) Scardino reported 5/8 patients with residual prostate cancer post-irradiation who experienced a complete response defined by negative follow-up biopsies.(16) We have also treated 2 patients with recurrent prostate cancer, both of whom responded. Wallace et al. have reported 9/15 patients who responded to IACP for advanced bladder cancer.(14) Sessions reported 2/4 patients with adenoidcystic cancers. Salem described responses in 2/3 patients with breast cancer metastatic to the liver, which confirms preliminary data published in Calvo's initial report of 9 patients with breast cancer.(13,15,6) In our own series (Table 1) we found 7/9 patients with primary hepatomas and 9/16 patients with metastatic adenocarcinoma of the lung to brain and liver who responded to IACP.

DISCUSSION

This series of clinical trials indicates that IACP is associated with a marked increase in therapeutic activity compared to intravenous cis-platinum in a wide spectrum of cancers. It must be concluded that arterial infusion of cis-platinum provides a significant pharmacologic advantage over intravenous cis-platinum, which could relate to the availability of active or unbound drug. These observations are in contrast to those of tumors that by comparison are exquisitively sensitive to intravenous cis-platinum, such as testicular and ovarian carcinomas, where high response rates can be achieved by intravenous infusion including 24-hour and 5-day drug administration schedules. There is now convincing clinical evidence of increased therapeutic activity for IACP in at léast 5 different tumor systems, including melanoma, sarcoma, head and neck cancers, colon cancer, and malignant gliomas. There is also preliminary data supporting the same observation for several other tumor systems including gynecological and bladder tumors, prostate cancer, breast cancer, adenoidcystic carcinomas, hepatomas and metastatic lung cancers. It would therefore appear that there is some as yet undefined, unique pharmacologic factor which gives IACP its therapeutic advantage.

The biological distribution and excretion of cis-platinum has been thoroughly studied.[21] The patterns of cis-platinum distribution, localization and excretion have been remarkably similar for several species, including rats, dogs, and man. Prehydration and diuresis with mannitol, furosemide, hypertonic saline or treatment with sodium thiosulfate do not alter plasma clearance or urinary excretion rates.[22,23] However, rate of infusion does significantly alter the urinary excretion pattern with a significantly smaller per cent excreted in patients receiving 24-hour cis-platinum infusions.[22] Cis-platinum has been shown to be rapidly and irreversibly bound to both protein and nonprotein plasma constituents and to the tissues.[24] Patients receiving cis-platinum as a 20-hour infusion have no detectable unbound cis-platinum during or following infusion, while patients receiving cis-platinum as a 1-hour infusion have unbound cis-platinum detectable for up to 1½ hours with a $T_{\frac{1}{2}}$ of approximately 45 to 60 minutes.[22] It is presumed that tissue binding ultimately takes the form of DNA binding, which is felt to represent the cytotoxic mechanism of action of cis-platinum.[22] Subcellular binding studies to date are incomplete. As previously noted, there have been many drug administration schedules primarily designed to reduce toxicity utilized for cis-platinum. There

There has been no evidence that therapeutic activity has been affected by drug administration schemas other than those already described for IACP administration.

Clinical pharmacologic studies comparing IACP and intravenous cis-platinum do not provide an explanation for the increased therapeutic activity observed for IACP.[25,26] However, preliminary, pharmacokinetic studies using a rat model system have demonstrated that the therapeutic activity of IACP infusion is influenced both by rate of infusion, with reduced efficacy at both too rapid and too slow an infusion time, and improved therapeutic efficacy using intraarterial occlusion, with consequent restricted hemodilution of drug during infusion.[27] This, in addition to the high response rate for intravenous cis-platinum in some tumor systems such as testicular cancers, suggests that active, perhaps unbound, drug availability and the specific tumor cell accessibility to active drug are important parameters in the mechanism of action of cis-platinum. The observed increased therapeutic activity for IACP, described in this review, make this the preferred route of administration when clinically feasible.

REFERENCES

1. Cvitkovic, E., Spaulding, J., Bethune, V., Martin, J., Whitmore, W.: Improvement of Cis-Dichlorodiammineplatinum. (NSC 119875). Therapeutic Index in an Animal Model. Cancer (39): 1357-1361. 1977.
2. Howell, S.B., Pfeifle, C.E., Wung, W.E., et al.: Intra-peritoneal Cisplatin with Systemic Thiosulfate Protection. Annals of Int. Med., (97): 845-851. 1982.
3. Ozols, R.F., Corden, B.J., Collins, J., Young, R.C.: High Dose Cisplatin in Hypertonic Saline: Renal Effects and Pharmacokinetics of a 40 MG/M^2 QD x 5 Schedule. In Platinum Coordination Complexes in Cancer Chemotherapy. Martinus Nijhoff Publishing, Boston, Mass. 1984. pp. 321-329.
4. Gralla, R., Itri, L., Pisko, S., Squillante, A., Kelsen, D., Braun, D., Bordin, L., Braun, T., Young, C.: Antiemetic with Placebo and Prochlorperazine in Patients with Chemo-therapy Induced Nausea & Vomiting: NEJM (305), 905-909. 1981.
5. Hydes, P.C., : Synthesis and Testing of Platinum Analogues An Overview. In Platinum Coordination Complexes in Cancer Chemotherapy. Martinus Nijhoff Publishing, Boston, Mass. 1984. pp. 216-227.
6. Calvo, D.B., Patt, Y.Z., Wallace, S., Chuang, V.P., Benjamin, R.S., Pritchard, J.D., Hersh, E.M., Bodey, G.P., Mavligit, G.M.: Phase I-II Trial of Percutaneous Intra-Arterial Cis-Diamminedichloroplatinum (II) for Regionally Confined Malignancy. Cancer (45), 1278-1283. 1980.
7. Pritchard, J.D., Mavligit, G.M., Benjamin, R.S., Patt, Y.Z., Calvo, D.B., Hall, S.W., Bodey, G.P., Wallace, S.: Regression of Regionally Confined Melanoma with Intra-Arterial Cis-Dichlorodiammineplatinum (II): Cancer Treatment Reports (63) 555-558. 1979.
8. Mavligit, G., Benjamin, R., Patt, Y., Jaffe, N., Chuang, V., Wallace, S., Murray, J., Ayala, A., Johnston, S., Hersh, E.M., Calvo, D.B.: Intraarterial Cis-Platinum for Patients with Inoperable Skeletal Tumors. Cancer (48) 1-4, 1981.
9. Lehane, D.E., Sessions, R., Johnson, P., Gomez, L., Horowitz, B., Bryan, R.N., DeSantos, L., Zubler, M.A., Durrance, F.Y.: Intra-Arterial Cis-Platinum in Head and Neck Cancer: Controlled Clinical Trial in Phases I and II. The International Head and Neck Oncology Research Conf. 1980.
10. Carlson, J., Freedman, R., Wallace, S., Chuang, V., Taylor Wharton, J., Rutledge, F.: Intraarterial Cis-Platinum in the Management of Squamous Cell Carcinoma of the Uterine Cervix. Gynecol. Oncol. (12) 92-98. 1981.
11. Lehane, D.E., Zubler, M.A., Lane, M., Smith, F.: Intra-Arterial Cisplatin in Metastatic or Recurrent Colon Cancer: Proceedings, Amer. Soc. of Clin. Onc. (12) 22, 1982.

12. Lehane, D.E., Bryan, R.N., Horowitz, B., DeSantos, L., Ehni, G., Zubler, M.A., Moiel, R., Rudolph, L., Aldama-Leubbert, A., Mahoney, D., Harper, R.: Intra-Arterial Cis-Platinum Chemotherapy for Patients with Primary and Metastatic Brain Tumors. Cancer Drug Delivery (1) 69-77. 1983.
13. Sessions, R.B., Lehane, D.E., Smith, R.J.H., Bryan, R.N., Suen, J.Y.: Intra-Arterial Cisplatin Treatment of Adenoid Cystic Carcinoma. Arch. Otol. (108) 221-224. 1982.
14. Wallace, S., Chuang, V.P., Samuels, M., Johnson, D.: Transcatheter Intraarterial Infusion of Chemotherapy in Advanced Bladder Cancer: Cancer (49) 640-645. 1982.
15. Salem, P.A., Khalil, M., Rizk, G., Jabboury, K., Hashimi, L.: Intra-Hepatic Artery Infusional Chemotherapy with Cis-Platinum in the Treatment of Metastatic Liver from Breast Cancer: Clinical Investigations. AACR. 191. 1981.
16. Scardino, P.T., Mata, J.A., Cantini, M.: Intra-Arterial Cisplatin (IA-DDP): Therapy for Radiorecurrent Carcinoma of the Prostate. Proceedings Amer. Urol. Assoc. 1984.
17. Steward, D.J., Wallace, S., Feun, L., Leavens, M., Young, S.E., Handel, S., Mavligit, G., Benjamin, R.S.: A Phase I Study of Intracarotid Artery Infusion of Cis-Diammine-dichloroplatinum (II) In Patients with Recurrent Malignant Intracerebral Tumors: Cancer Research (42) 2059-2062. 1982.
18. Kovach, J., Moertel, C., Schutt, A., Reitmeier, R., Hahn, R. Phase II Study of Cis-Diamminedichloroplatinum (NSC 119875) in Advanced Carcinoma of the Large Bowel: Cancer Chemotherapy Reports (57) 357-359. 1973.
19. Lavin, P., Mittelman, A., Douglass, H., Engstrom, P., Klassen, D.: Survival & Response to Chemotherapy for Advanced Colorectal Adenocarcinoma. Cancer (46) 1536-1543. 1980.
20. Walker, M., Green, S., Byar, D., Alexander, E., Betzdorf, U., Brooks, W., Hunt, W., MacCarthy, C., Mahaley, M., Mealey, J., Owens, G., RansHoff, J., Robertson, J., Shapiro, W., Smith, K., Wilson, C., Strike, T.: Randomized Comparisons of Radiotherapy and Nitrosoureas for the Treatment of Malignant Glioma after Surgery. NEJM (303) 1323-1329. 1980.
21. Taylor, D.: The Pharmacokinetics of Cis-Diamminedichloroplatinum (II) in Animals and Man: Relation to Treatment Scheduling. Biochimie (60) 949-956. 1978.
22. Himmelstein, K., Patton, T., Belt, R., Taylor, S., Repeta, A., Stevenson, L.: Clinical Kinetics of Intact Cis-Platin and Some Related Species. Clin. Pharm. Ther. (29) 658-664. 1981
23. Howell, S.B., Pfeifle, C.E., Wung, W.E. et al.: Intra-Peritoneal Cis-Diamminedichloroplatinum with Systemic Thiosulfate Protection. Canc. Res. (43) 1426-1431, 1983.
24. Cole, W.C., Wolf, W.: Preparation and Metabolism of a Cis-Platin/Serum Protein Complex. Chem. Biol. Interactions. (30) 223-235. 1980.

25. Stewart, D.J., Benjamin, R.S., Zimmerman, S., Caprioli, R.M., Wallace, S., Chuang, V., Calvo, D., Samuels, M., Bonura, J., Loo, R.L.: Clinical Pharmacology of Intra-Arterial Cis-Diamminedichloroplatinum (II). Canc. Res. (43) 917-920. 1983.
26. Campbell, T.N., Howell, S.B., Pfeifle, C.E., Wung, W.E., Bookstein, J.: Clinical Pharmacokinetics of Intraarterial Cisplatin in Humans: Journal of Clin. Oncol. (1) 755-762. 1983.
27. Lehane, D.E., Lane, M., Busch, H.: Intra-Arterial Cis-Platinum (IACP), A Rat Model for Pharmacokinetic Studies: In Platinum Coordination Complexes in Cancer Chemotherapy. Martinus Nijhoff Publ., Boston, Mass. 1984. p. 142.

HEPATIC ARTERIAL INFUSION OF FLOXURIDINE, ADRIAMYCIN, AND MITOMYCIN C FOR PRIMARY LIVER NEOPLASMS

Yehuda Z.Patt, M.D., Chusilp Charnsangavej, M.D., and Marilyn Soski, R.N.

INTRODUCTION

Survival of untreated patients with inoperable primary liver neoplasms is approximately 75 days (1,2). Before Adriamycin, both intravenous and intra-arterial chemotherapeutic agents had very little effect upon the survival of these patients despite tumor shrinkage (3,4). Adriamycin given IV as a single agent or in combination with other drugs resulted initially in a response of 78% (5). Later studies reported response rates ranging from 9% to 44% (6-14). In 67% of patients with primary liver neoplasms, disease seems confined to the liver at the time of diagnosis, and even at autopsy disease is still confined to the liver in 44% of the patients (15). A regional approach to a disease with such dismal prognosis seems warranted. A pilot study of hepatic arterial infusion of floxuridine, Adriamycin, and mitomycin C (FUDRAM) resulted in a response rate of 66% in patients with hepatocellular carcinoma (16). We decided, therefore, to explore this treatment regimen further.

MATERIAL AND METHODS

Forty-four patients with primary hepatic neoplasms were treated according to this regimen. Their clinical characteristics are described in Table 1.

TABLE 1. PRETREATMENT PROGNOSTIC FACTORS

Characteristic	Hepatoma	Cholangio-carcinoma	Unknown Primary
Evaluable Pts.	30	6	8
Sex (M-F ratio)	19:11	3:3	3:5
*Age (yr)	53.5	53	51
Range	(21 - 70))	(40 - 68)	(28 - 75)
Race (W:B:O:L)	19:2:4:5	6:0:0:0	8:0:0:0)
PS*	2	1	2
Range	(0 - 3)	(0 - 2)	(0 - 3)
AFP* (ng/ml)	247.5	17.6	14.1
Range	(5.5 - 122,400)	(8.8 - 37.4)	(2.3 - 371.2)
CEA* (ng/ml)	6.75	38.4	25.8
Range	(1.5 - 31.8)	(4.8 - 375.3)	(5.9 - 71.0)
Bilirubin* (mg/dl)	0.7	1.05	0.6
Range	(0.3 - 30.4)	(0.2 - 17.4)	(0.2 - 2.1)
SAP*	265	197	>350
Range	(97 - >350)	(147 - >350)	(108 - >350)

*Median. Abbreviations: W = white, B = black, O = oriental, L = latin, PS = Performance status, AFP = Alphafetoprotein, CEA = Carcinoembryonic antigen, SAP = Serum Alkaline phosphatase

Thirty patients had primary hepatocellular carcinoma, six had cholangiocarcinoma, seven had unidentified primaries, and one had pancreatic cancer. These eight patients were included together under the heading "unknown primary". Sex ratio, ages, racial composition, performance status, and pretreatment levels of alpha-fetoprotein (AFP), carcinoembryonic antigen (CEA), bilirubin, and serum alkaline phosphatase (SAP) are also shown in Table 1.

Catheters were inserted percutaneously into the hepatic artery by the Seldinger technique before each course of chemotherapy, i.e., every 4 to 5 weeks; intervals between courses depended on the degree of myelosuppression or stomatitis resulting from the preceding course. The femoral approach was employed for inserting the arterial catheter. One course of chemotherapy consisted of the following: Adriamycin, 40 mg/m^2, was mixed in 200 ml of 5% dextrose in one-half normal saline and administered over 2 hours (the dose had to be reduced to as low as 10 mg/m^2 in patients with jaundice); mitomycin C, 10 mg/m^2, was mixed in 400 ml of normal saline supplemented with 1000 units of heparin and infused over 2 hours. This was followed by daily administration of 75 mg/m^2 of floxuridine (FUDR) mixed in 1000 ml of 5% dextrose in one-fourth normal saline and supplemented with 15000 units of heparin (Table 2).

TABLE 2. HEPATIC ARTERIAL INFUSION OF FUDR, ADRIAMYCIN AND MITOMYCIN C (FUDRAM) FOR THE TREATMENT OF PRIMARY LIVER NEOPLASMS

Treatment Plan*			
Agent	Days	Dose (mg/m^2)	Mode of Administration
FUDR	1 - 5	75	Continuous 5-day infusion
Adriamycin**	1	10 - 40	2-hour infusion
Mitomycin	1	10	2-hour infusion

*Percutaneous catheterizations and treatment repeated every 4-6 weeks.
** Adriamycin dose was decreased in jaundiced patients.

FUDR was given by continuous infusion over 5 days. Chemotherapy was administered with an IMED 922 volumetric infusion pump (IMED Corp., San Diego, CA), as previously described (17-19). At the end of each infusion cycle (usually on day 6), the catheter was removed.

Tumor response was evaluated by radionuclide liver scanning, sonography, computerized tomography, and hepatic angiography, all collectively termed "imaging techniques" and supplemented by concomitant serial measurements of serum AFP in patients with hepatocellular tumors and by serum CEA in those with the unknown primary tumors or cholangiocarcinoma. A complete remission (CR) was defined as complete disappearance of all evidence of existing tumor as determined by the techniques listed above and return of AFP or CEA to normal values. A partial response (PR) was defined as $\geq$50% reduction in the size of the tumor as measured by a product of the two largest perpendicular diameters of each of the tumor masses, along with a decrease of $\geq$50% in AFP or CEA. A shrinkage of <50% in tumor size and a decrease of <50% in AFP or CEA was defined as a response of <PR. Duration of response was calculated from the time tumor dimension decreased by $\geq$50% in the imaging tests or a decrease of $\geq$50% was observed in the AFP or CEA to the time either measurement had returned to preresponse levels.

Estimated curves for survival were plotted from the first day of treatment by the method of Kaplan and Meier, (20), and statistical significance of differences was determined according to Gehan's modification of the generalized Wilcoxon test (21).

RESULTS

Treatment results are described in Table 3.

TABLE 3. RESPONSE TO HEPATIC ARTERIAL INFUSION OF FUDRAM

Type of Response	Hepatoma	Cholangio Ca	Unknown 1°	Total
CR	3 (10%)	1	0	4
PR	18 (60%)	1	0	19
CR + PR	(70%)	(33.3%)		(52.2%)
No Change	3 (10%)	1 (16.6%)	2 (25%)	6
Progression	4 (13.3%)	2 (33.3%)	4 (50%)	10
Total	30	6	8	44

Thus, among patients with hepatoma, three complete remissions and 18 partial remissions were observed, for a response rate of 70%. In addition, two patients (6.6%) experienced a response of <PR. Three hepatoma patients had no change in their disease (10%), and four progressed while on treatment (13.3%). Of six patients with cholangiocarcinoma, one patient had a CR and one a PR for a response rate of 33%. None of the eight patients with unknown primary tumors in the liver had a response. Two patients had <PR. Over-all, a response rate of 52% was observed among these 44 patients with hepatic arterial infusion of FUDRAM. A representative pretreatment hepatic arteriogram of a patient with hepatoma is shown in Figure 1.

FIGURE 1. PRETREATMENT HEPATIC ARTERIOGRAM.

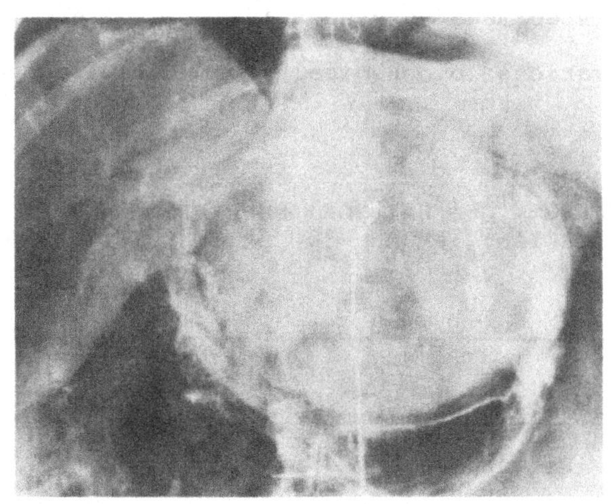

FIGURE 2. FOLLOW-UP ARTERIOGRAM IN THE SAME PATIENT AFTER 1 TREATMENT CYCLE.

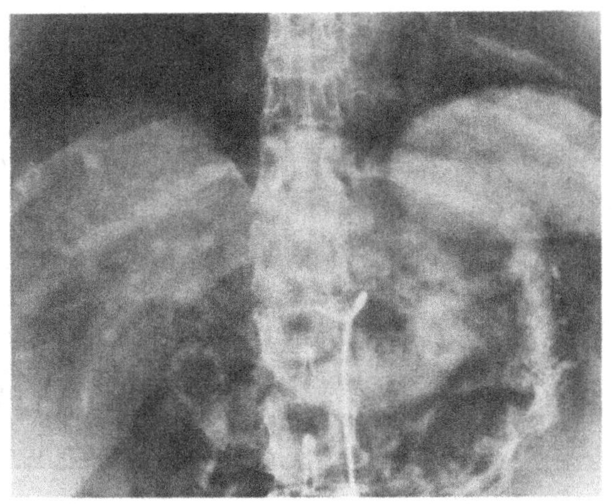

This patient's tumor eventually completely disappeared. Second-look surgery at 12 months failed to show any residual disease in the liver, and results from studies of multiple liver biopsy specimens were negative. The effects of HAI of FUDRAM on various biochemical parameters are summarized in table 4.

TABLE 4. EFFECT OF HAI OF FUDRAM ON SOME BIOCHEMICAL PARAMETERS (MEDIAN) AMONG 30 PATIENTS WITH HEPATOCELLULAR CARCINOMA

PARAMETER		PRE		POST
AFP ng/ml	Responders (range)	247.5 (2.5 - 122400)	**	24.8 (1.3 - 13600)
	Nonresponders (range)	380.9 (196 - 63200)		538.5 (62.4 - 56000)
CEA ng/ml	Responders (range)	7.1 (1.5 - 31.8)		7.3 (1.5 - 14.5)
	Nonresponders (range)	6.4 (1.5 - 9.1)		5.0 (1.5 - 10.6)
Bilirubin mg/dl	Responders (range)	.7 (.3 - 30.4)	*	.4 (.2 - 1.8)
	Nonresponders (range)	.8 (.5 - 10)		.5 (.5 - 26)
Alkaline Phosphatase mu/ml	Responders (range)	237 (97 - >350)	*	145 (72 - >350)
	Nonresponders (range)	>350 (194 - >350)	*	203 (106 - >350)

* P<.05
** P<.01

Median AFP among responding patients was 247.5 ng/ml and dropped to 24.8 (P.<.01), and among nonresponders the respective values were 280.9 and 538.5 ng/ml. The median bilirubin level dropped from .7 to .4 mg/dl (P<.05). In one patient a pretreatment bilirubin level of 30.4 mg/dl returned to 0.9 mg/dl, and in another patient the bilirubin level dropped from 5.7 to 0.8 ng/dl in response to treatment. Median response duration was 5 months. Median survival among all hepatoma patients was 11.2 months from diagnosis and 8.2 months from treatment.

Responding hepatoma patients (CR, PR, and <PR) had a median survival of 10 months from beginning of treatment, as opposed to only 4.0 months among the non-responders (P=.03) (Figure 3).

FIGURE 3.

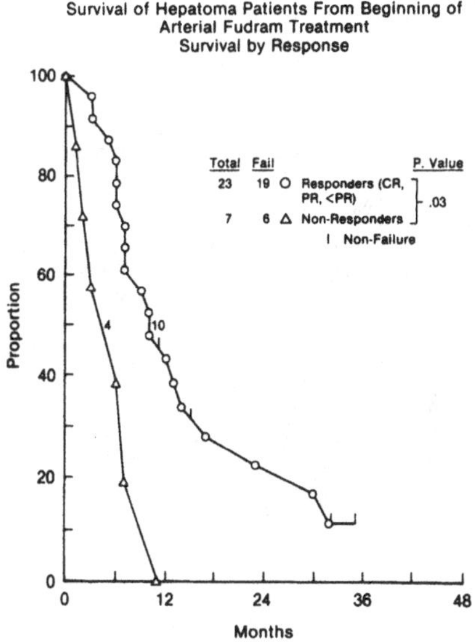

Prolonged survival was seen in five of the responding patients whose tumors became resectable following hepatic arterial FUDRAM. They survived 35+, 32+, 11+, 11+ and 30 months from the initiation of arterial therapy (Table 5). The last patient relapsed in the liver after being off treatment for 18 months. She refused to resume treatment. Median survival among nonhepatoma patients was 8.8 months from diagnosis and 7.9 months from treatment. Only two of six cholangiocarcinoma patients and none of the patients with unknown primary liver neoplasms responded to the treatment. Median survival from diagnosis among three hepatoma patients with a Zubrod's performance status of 0 has not been reached but will exceed 19 months. It was 11.6 months among 18 patients with a Zubrod's performance status of 1-2 and 6.0 months among eight patients with a Zubrod's performance status of 3 (Figure 4).

FIGURE 4.

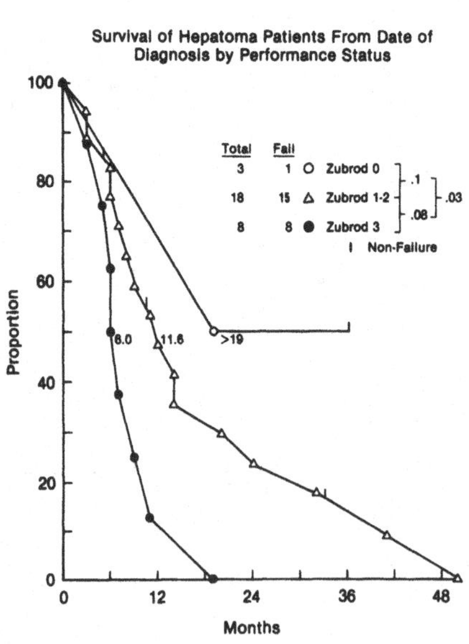

The respective survival data from treatment were 17.0 months, 10.6 months, and 6.0 months. Arterial occlusion was effected in 10 of the 30 hepatoma patients. Survival was not significantly longer in those with arterial occlusion (11.6 vs. 7.0 months in those without occlusion, P=.18). Chemotherapy-related complications observed in patients treated with hepatic arterial infusion of FUDRAM are summarized in Table 5.

TABLE 5. CHEMOTHERAPY RELATED COMPLICATIONS ASSOCIATED WITH HEPATIC ARTERIAL INFUSION (HAI) OF FUDRAM

Side-Effect	Incidence
Anemia (<8.0 gm/100 ml hemoglobin)	22.7
Granulocytopenia (<10 AGC)	22.7
Thrombocytopenia (<75,000 platelets)	22.7
Alopecia*	100.0
Nausea and Vomiting	9.0
Dyspepsia	9.0
Gastritis	4.5
Diarrhea	6.8
Mucositis	11.3
Transient Renal Failure	2.2

Abbreviation: AGC = Absolute granulocyte count.
*Alopecia occurred in all patients after more than two cycles.

Thus, anemia, granulocytopenia, and thrombocytopenia were each observed in 23.6% of the cycles. Alopecia was observed in all patients treated with hepatic arterial infusion of FUDRAM. Nausea, vomiting, dyspepsia, gastritis, diarrhea, and mucositis all occurred with the incidences shown in table 5. Transient renal failure was associated with the high volume of contrast medium used during angiography.

DISCUSSION

The results of this study demonstrate the efficacy of FUDRAM in patients with primary liver neoplasms. Thus, hepatic arterial infusion of FUDRAM resulted in a response rate of 70% and a median survival of 10 months among responders and only 4 months among nonresponding patients with hepatoma. Among patients with cholangiocarcinoma, a response rate of 33.3% was observed. Hepatic arterial infusion of FUDRAM was of no benefit in the management of unknown primary neoplasms in the liver. The high response rate associated with this treatment is particularly interesting in view of the fact that intravenous adriamycin or Adriamycin-containing chemotherapy combinations resulted in a response rate of only 9%-40% (5-14). A possibility exists that a fluoropyrimidine, Adriamycin, and mitomycin C regimen given IV would have also produced a high response rate and prolonged survival. However, administration of all three agents by the hepatic arterial route resulted in an increased hepatic extraction ratio ranging from 100 to

400-fold for FUDR (22), and 3 to 5-fold for mitomycin C (23), and 2-fold for Adriamycin (24). This suggests that increased response and survival were associated with the increased drug concentration gradient resulting from the arterial route of administration and a possible synergism between the three agents. Falkson et al. (25), when analyzing survival from diagnosis among North American patients in reference to their respective performance statuses, found a median survival of 52 weeks for those with Zubrod's 0 performance status, 18 weeks for those with a Zubrod's 1-2 performance status, and 5 weeks for those with a Zubrod's 3 performance status. Our treatment resulted in median survival of >19 months, 11.6 months, and 6 months in patients with these respective performance statuses.

Despite these encouraging results, only patients who achieved a CR or whose residual liver disease could be surgically resected enjoyed prolonged survival. All others whose disease was not completely eradicated by chemotherapy or surgery eventually relapsed. To achieve optimal palliation in this latter group of patients, one should consider the use of an Infusaid-type implantable arterial infusion device to facilitate continued long-term therapy. In one patient who failed to respond to HAI of FUDRAM, additional palliation in terms of antitumor response and prolongation of survival was achieved by utilizing the ischemic effects of arterial embolization combined with cisplatin particles at a dose of 100 mg/m^2. Extrahepatic disease developed in ten of the hepatoma patients and contributed to the demise of four of them.

Arterial infusion of FUDRAM can thus offer palliation, prolongation of survival, and in some cases long-term survival in patients with hepatocellular carcinoma who could achieve a chemotherapy-induced or surgical CR. This treatment had, however, only a marginal effect upon patients with cholangiocarcinoma and none upon patients with unknown primary tumors metastatic to the liver. Drugs such as cisplatin or cisplatinum combined with etoposide (13) could possibly be used in nonhepatoma patients or in hepatoma patients failing HAI of FUDRAM.

REFERENCES

1. Purves LR, Bersohn I, Geddes EW: Serum alpha fetoprotein and primary cancer of the liver in man. Cancer (25):1261-1270, 1970.
2. Jaffe BM, Donegan WL, Watson, S, Spratt JS: Factors influencing survival in patients with untreated hepatic metastases. Surg Gynecol Obstet (128):1-11, 1975.
3. Moertel GC: Clinical management of advanced gastrointestinal cancer. Cancer (36):675-682, 1975.
4. Al-Sarraf M, Go TS, Kithier K, Vaitkevicius ZK: Primary liver cancer: A review of the clinical features, blood groups, serum enzymes, therapy and survival of 65 cases. Cancer (33):574-582, 1974.
5. Olweny CLM, Toya T, Katongole-Mbidde E, Mugerwa J, Kyalwazi SK, Cohen H: Treatment of hepatocellular carcinoma with adriamycin. Cancer (36) 1250-1257, 1975.
6. Vogel CL, Bayley AC, Brooker RJ, Anthony PP, Ziegler JL: A phase II study of adriamycin (NSC 123127) in patients with hepatocellular carcinoma from Zambia and the United States. Cancer (39):1923-1929, 1977.
7. Baker LH, Saiki JH, Jones SE, Hewlett JS, Brownlee RW, Stephens RL, Vaitkevicius VK: Adriamycin and 5-Fluorouracil in the treatment of advanced hepatoma: A Southwest Oncology Group. Cancer Treat Rep (61): 1595-1597, 1977.
8. Falkson G, Moertel CG, Lavin P, Pretorius FJ, Carbone PP: Chemotherapy studies in primary liver cancer. A

prospective randomized clinical trial. Cancer (42):2149-2156, 1978.
9. Johnson PJ, Williams R, Thomas H, Sherlock S, Murray-Lyon IM: Induction of remission in hepatocellular carcinoma with doxorubicin. Lancet (1):1006-1009, 1978.
10. Vilaseca J, Guardia J, Bacardi R, Monne J: Doxorubicin for liver cancer. Lancet (1):1367, 1978.
11. Olweny CLM, Katongole-Mbidde E, Bahendeka S, Otim D, Mugerwa J, Kyalwazi SK: Further experience in treating patients with hepatocellular carcinoma in Uganda. Cancer (46):2717-2722, 1980.
12. Morstyn G, Ihde DC, Eddy JL, Bunn PA, Cohen MH, Minna JD: Combination chemotherapy of hepatocellular carcinoma with doxorubicin and streptozotocin. Am J Clin Oncol (6):547-551, 1983.
13. Melia WM, Johnson PJ, Williams R: Induction of remission in hepatocellular carcinoma. Cancer (51):206-210, 1983.
14. Choi TK, Lee NW, Wong J: Chemotherapy for advanced hepatocellular carcinoma. Cancer (53):401-405, 1984.
15. Appelqvist P: Primary carcinoma of the liver: Clinical course and therapeutic results. J Surg Oncol (21):87-93, 1982.
16. Patt, YZ, Chuang VP, Wallace S, Benjamin RS, Fuqua R, Mavligit GM: Hepatic arterial chemotherapy and occlusion for palliation of primary hepatocellular and unknown primary neoplasms in the liver. Cancer (51):1359-1363, 1983.
17. Patt, YZ, Mavligit GM, Chuang VP, Wallace S, Johnston S, Benjamin RS, Valdivieso M, Hersh, EM: Percutaneous hepatic infusion (HAI) of mitomycin C and floxuridine (FUDR): An effective treatment for metastatic colorectal carcinoma in the liver. Cancer (46):261-265, 1980.
18. Patt, YZ , Chuang VP, Wallace S, Johnston S, Fuqua R, Hersh EM, Freireich EJ, Mavligit GM: The palliative role of hepatic arterial infusion and arterial occlusion in colorectal carcinoma metastatic to the liver. Lancet (1):349-351, 1981.
19. Patt, YZ, Peters RE, Chuang VP, Wallace S, Fuqua R, Mavligit GM: Effective retreatment of patients with colorectal cancer and liver metastases. Amer J Med (75):237-240, 1983.
20. Kaplan EL, Meier P: Non-parametric estimation from incomplete observation. J AM Stat Assoc (53):457-481, 1958.
21. Gehan EA: A generalized Wilcoxon test for comparing arbitrarily single censored samples. Biometrica (52):203-223, 1965.
22. Ensminger WD, Rosowsky A, Raso V, Lewin DC, Glode M, Come S, Steele G, Frei E III: A clinical pharmacological evaluation of hepatic arterial infusions of 5-fluoro-2'-deoxyuridine and 5-fluorouracil. Cancer Res (38):378-3792, 1978.
23. Gyves J, Ensimger W, Stetson P, VanHarken D, Janis M, Cho K, Meyer S, Walker S, Gilbertson S, Niederhuber J:

Clinical pharmacology of mitomycin C (Mito) by hepatic arterial (HA) infusion. Pro ASCO (2):C-97, 1983.
24. Garnick MB, Ensminger WD, Israel M: A clinical-pharmacological evaluation of hepatic arterial infusion of Adriamycin. Cancer Res (39):4105-4110, 1979.
25. Falkson G, McIntyre JM, Moertel CG, Johnson LA, Sherman RC: Primary liver cancer , an ECOG therapeutic trial. Cancer, in press 1984.

INTRAARTERIAL ADRIAMYCIN, RADIATION THERAPY, AND SURGICAL EXCISION FOR EXTREMITY SKELETAL AND SOFT-TISSUE SARCOMAS

F.R. EILBER, J. MIRRA, J. ECKARDT, D. KERN

1. INTRODUCTION

Local control of extremity soft-tissue sarcomas is still a significant and important clinical problem. Although surgical procedures have been extended from simple excisions to more radical and super-radical amputative procedures, the local recurrence rate for both the skeletal and soft-tissue sarcomas remains high and in most series approaches 20-30% if treatment is surgery alone (1-6). Because local recurrence of these highly malignant tumors usually foretells poor prognosis, the local control of these lesions becomes an important consideration. Megavoltage radiation therapy, the delivery of high doses of external beam radiation, just after the following surgical procedures has reduced the local recurrence rate to approximately 15-20% and improved the overall survival (7-9).

Adriamycin, 14-hydroxydaunomycin, was found to be an effective anti-tumor antibiotic for patients with the metastatic skeletal or soft-tissue sarcomas. The initial reports by Gottlieb et al. in the early 1970's showed an overall response rate of approximately 40% for tumors that previously were resistant to other known single chemotherapeutic agents (10). In addition to the well-known side effects of alopecia, cardiomyopsy, mucositis, and gastrointestinal toxicity, several investigators reported marked local toxicity from the infiltration of soft tissue during intravenous administration in the early clinical studies of Adriamycin (11). Marked tissue necrosis and augmented tumor "flair" was observed in patients who were also receiving radiation therapy (12).

In 1974, with this information in mind, we began a series of studies in which patients with extremity skeletal or soft-tissue sarcomas were treated with Adriamycin by intraarterial infusion (13-15). This paper will review our experiences with a consecutive series of these patients. Our purpose was to develop an effective preoperative protocol with a combination of intraarterial Adriamycin and subsequent radiation therapy to induce in vivo tumor-cell necrosis in an effort both to avoid amputative surgery and to reduce local tumor recurrence in patients with extremity skeletal or soft-tissue sarcomas.

2. MATERIALS AND METHODS

From 1973 to 1983, a total of 427 patients with extremity skeletal or soft-tissue sarcomas were evaluated by the Division of Surgical Oncology, UCLA School of Medicine. Of these, 163 were skeletal sarcomas and 264 were soft-tissue sarcomas. Two hundred ninety-three patients, or 68%, were entered into the prospective limb-salvage protocols. This was not a randomized trial, and patients were excluded from the protocols for low-grade sarcomas, for amputation performed prior to coming to UCLA, and, in a very small group, because of the tumor size (Table 1).

A complete history was taken on all patients, and physical and laboratory examinations included SMA-12, CBC, chest x-ray or lung tomograms, and, most recently, CAT scans of the chest and of the extremity. Histology of all lesions was confirmed by biopsy and examination by one of the authors, Dr. Mirra.

Preoperative Adriamycin was administered by an indwelling arterial catheter placed by percutaneous puncture of either the femoral or brachial artery using the Seldinger technique. Catheters were positioned in the axillary artery for upper extremity lesions and in the common femoral artery for lower

Table 1. Extremity Sarcoma — UCLA (1973-1983)

	Total Seen	Protocol IA Adria, XRT, Surgery
Sarcoma Extremity	472	293 (68%)
Skeletal	163	103 (63%)
Soft Tissue	264	190 (72%)

extremity lesions. For the proximal thigh lesions or buttock lesions, the catheters were positioned in either the internal or external iliac artery. Routine arteriograms evaluated tumor blush and vascular displacement. Drug distribution was monitored by injections of fluorescein dye and a Woods lamp. If the distribution of the dye varied from the primary tumor site, the catheters were repositioned until a proper distribution was obtained. Early in our experience, we based catheter placement on the tumor's arterial blood supply at the time of angiography only to find that this blood supply did not necessarily correlate with the drug-flow patterns of the vascular system demonstrated by fluorescein distribution.

Adriamycin was infused at a dosage of 30 mg in 500 ml of saline for lower extremity lesions and at 20 mg for lesions of the upper extremity. The infusate was delivered over a 24-hour period by an IVAC infusion pump for each of 3 consecutive days. Daily fluorescein dye injections confirmed proper catheter placement, but if hot spots or skin erythema were noted, the catheters were repositioned to change the distribution pattern.

Early in our experience, the catheters were placed in the superficial femoral or popliteal artery for distal lesion or into the brachial artery for forearm lesions. Severe complications, such as erythema of the skin and fibrosis of the subcutaneous tissue, occurred until we realized that the catheters were approximately the same size as the vessel being infused and in many instances acted as a perfusion rather than infusion with this high drug dose. Subsequently, catheters were placed in high-flow vessels. Heparin was also added to the system in the first three patients, but it was clear that it caused precipitation of the Adriamycin, and it was discontinued.

At the completion of the 72-hour infusion, the catheter was removed, and manual pressure was placed on the artery before external beam radiation therapy with a Cobalt 60 generator was given from 1 to a maximum of 4 days. Radiation was delivered through AP-PA ports to a dose range of 350 R times 10 for 139 patients and 350 R fractions times 5 for 164 patients. The entire anatomic region, i.e. thigh or calf, was treated, except for a strip of skin opposite the biopsy site. All radiation therapy was performed on an outpatient basis.

Surgical excision of the involved lesion took place from 3-6 weeks following the completion of the preoperative therapy. All surgical procedures included the previous biopsy scar in continuity with the tumor resection. Operations were performed through uninvolved tissue planes with pathologic confirmation of negative margins. For the soft-tissue sarcomas, excision was extended to include the adventitia of adjacent blood vessels or perineurium of major nerves in the vicinity of the tumor as well as a cuff of normal tissue. Furthermore, if a soft-tissue tumor was intimately associated with the periosteum, the periosteum was removed. For the skeletal sarcomas, the procedure involved *en bloc* excision of the diseased bone and adjacent muscle, with a bony margin of 10 cm proximal to all gross x-ray and scan evidence of tumor extension. The intermedullary canal was curetted for pathologic confirmation of a negative proximal or distal marrow. Twenty-three patients had diseased bone replaced by cadaver allografts, and 75 received metallic endoprostheses. Twenty-six patients required no bony replacement, 13 of whom had an internal pelvectomy without support for the lesions of the hemipelvis or a portion thereof.

Excised tumor specimens were examined by Dr. Mirra. At least 15 sections were taken from the surgical margin and the central portion of each tumor. An estimation of tumor-cell necrosis was based on the lack of nuclei. All 15 slides of each specimen were examined by at least 10 high-power fields per sample. Estimates of tumor-cell necrosis were based on a percentage of the total tumor mass.

Clonogenic assays were performed on 200 specimens, not only to evaluate the visual tumor-cell necrosis and the ability or inability of the tumor, but to test for drug sensitivity. The clonogenic assays were performed by the method of Salmon, with modifications previously described by Kern (16,17). A total of 215 sarcoma specimens were processed, and 106 were successfully tested for in vitro chemosensitivity, an overall success rate of 49%. In vitro sensitivity, defined as less than 50% colony formation, showed that the active single chemotherapeutic agents were Adriamycin (30.3), cis-Platinum (28.9%), and Cytoxan (31.7%) (Melphalan or L-PAM because Cytoxin is inactive in vitro). In vitro/in vivo correlations were possible in 34 sarcoma patients. Six patients whose tumors were sensitive in vitro to at least one anticancer drug were treated with that drug, and three of the six had a favorable clinical response of at least a 50% reduction in measurable tumor. The other three patients showed no evidence of clinical benefit. Twenty-four of 28 patients whose tumors were resistant to drug in vitro showed no clinical response, and four patients responded to a drug to which their tumor was resistant in vitro.

The various limb-salvage protocols and the number of patients treated in each group are shown in Table 2. The pilot study of 10 patients indicated that local excision of the tumor could be performed in five, but that amputation was necessary in the other five. No radiation therapy was given to these patients, and they only received preoperative intraarterial Adriamycin.

Table 2. Limb-Salvage Protocols — UCLA.

Year	Protocol	# Patients
1. 1973-1974	IA Adriamycin, Surgery	10
2. 1974-1981	IA Adriamycin, 3500 R, Surgery	139
3. 1981-1983	IA Adriamycin, 1750 R, Surgery	164
4. 1984-	IA Adriamycin vs. IV Adriamycin, 1750 R, Surgery	

Evaluation of tumor-cell necrosis showed that 40% of the 10 tumors were necrotic by pathologic criteria.

It was evident that intraarterial Adriamycin had some effect on these tumors, even though additional therapy was necessary. Therefore, the next 139 patients were treated by the identical intraarterial Adriamycin dose, followed by 3500 R of radiation to the tumor. Of these 139 patients, 82 had extremity soft-tissue sarcomas, and 56 had extremity skeletal sarcomas, 90% of which were osteosarcoma. Amputation was necessary for 1/56 patients with skeletal sarcoma and for 2/82 with soft-tissue sarcoma. Local tumor failure occurred in two skeletal sarcoma patients and in three with soft-tissue sarcoma, for a local control rate of 97%. The overall survival rate for patients with soft-tissue sarcoma was 70% at 5 years, and for the high-grade bone tumors was 56% at 5 years.

Significant complications related to the preoperative therapy occurred in the soft-tissue sarcoma group. Arterial thrombosis occurred in two patients early in the series. The thrombosis has not been seen after placement of the catheters in the high-flow vessels. One of these patients subsequently required amputation, even though a bypass was attempted, and the other required embolectomy.

Table 3. Soft-Tissue Sarcomas — Complications of Treatment (IA Adriamycin, Radiation)

	Number = 82			
	3500 R		1750 R	
Complications	27	32%	19	17%
Wound Slough	14	17%	17	15%
Fracture	7	9%	2	2%
Edema	4	5%	2	2%

Twenty-seven complications (32%) occurred in patients with the soft-tissue sarcomas who received 3500 R radiation. Complications included wound slough in 17%, lymphedema in 5%, and subsequent fracture of an adjacent long bone approximately 1-2 years later (Table 3). This 9% incidence of fracture was not anticipated, and all were treated by intramedullary rods after a biopsy showed no evidence of tumor recurrence. All have subsequently healed.

Because of this relatively high complication rate, a third protocol was developed that included intraarterial Adriamycin but reduced the radiation by half to 1750 R before surgical excision. One hundred sixty-four patients have been treated by this protocol — 108 with extremity soft-tissue sarcoma and 55 with skeletal sarcoma. Limb salvage has been possible in the same number of patients as the second trial, in that amputation was required for three with soft-tissue sarcoma and for one with skeletal sarcoma. The local recurrence rate has been equally low — one local recurrence in the skeletal sarcoma group and three in the soft-tissue group. Pathologic evidence of tumor-cell necrosis has been equal in the bone tumors but has changed for the soft-tissue sarcomas (Table 4). The amount of necrosis achieved by intraarterial Adriamycin/radiation therapy was grade-related in that Grade I tumors had very little necrosis,

Table 4. Soft-Tissue Sarcomas — Pathologic Tumor Necrosis (IA Adriamycin & Radiation)

3500 R				1750 R			
		Path Necrosis				Path Necrosis	
Grade	N	Range	Median	Grade	N	Range	Median
I	1	10	10%	I	1	5	5%
II	11	(10-90)	50%	II	25	(10-80)	25%
III	70	(10-100)	80%	III	82	(10-100)	50%
	82				108		

Grade II had an intermediate amount, and Grade III had the highest. Necrosis decreased approximately 25% for each grade by decreasing the radiation dose from 1750 to 350%. Thus far, this change has not translated into a higher local recurrence rate.

The complication rate has been reduced, however, from 32% to 17%, or 19/108 patients with soft-tissue sarcomas. Wound slough is still the most common problem and has remained relatively constant at 15%. Fractures have been reduced to 2%, as has lymphedema.

Limb salvage has been achieved in 93% of the patients with skeletal sarcoma, and amputation has only been necessary for 2/103 consecutive patients, or 7%. Limb salvage has been possible in 97% of patients with soft-tissue sarcoma. Amputation was required for only 5/190 consecutive patients. During the same time interval, of those patients with skeletal sarcoma who were not entered into the limb-salvage protocol and were treated either by surgery alone or surgery plus postoperative radiation, 34/60 (56%) required amputation, as did 19/74 (30%) with soft-tissue sarcomas. Again, this was not a randomized trial, and the amputation rate in the non-protocol patients was similar to that reported in the literature. The local tumor recurrence rate for the protocol patients

Table 5. Extremity Sarcoma: Amputation

	Limb Salvage	Non-Limb Salvage
Skeletal	2/103 (2%)	34/60 (57%)
Soft Tissue	5/190 (3%)	19/74 (26%)

Table 6. Extremity Sarcoma — Local Tumor Recurrence

	Limb Salvage	Non-Limb Salvage
Skeletal	3/103 (2%)	6/60 (10%)
Soft Tissue	6/190 (3%)	12/74 (16%)

(Table 5) was 3/103 (7%) for skeletal sarcoma and 6/190 (3%) for soft-tissue sarcomas. The non-limb-salvage group with skeletal sarcoma had a 10% local recurrence rate, and 16% for the 74 patients with soft-tissue sarcoma (Table 6).

3. DISCUSSION

This report summarizes our experience with intraarterial Adriamycin in 293 patients for extremity skeletal or soft-tissue sarcomas. Tumor-cell necrosis in 10 patients treated by intraarterial Adriamycin alone averaged 40%, and limb salvage was only possible in half of these patients. In a subsequent protocol of intraarterial Adriamycin and 3500 R of radiation followed by en bloc resection, among 139 patients, limb salvage was possible in 95%, and local tumor recurrence was kept to only 6%. However, with this protocol, there was a local complication rate of approximately 32%, and half of the patients involved required reoperation, with one amputation. A third protocol of intraarterial Adriamycin and 1750 R of radiation for 164 patients had an equal limb-salvage rate of 97%, low local tumor recurrence of 3%, and a complication rate of 17%. Evidence of tumor-cell destruction was reduced by approximately 25% in extremity soft-tissue sarcomas treated with a lower dose of radiation but was equal in the high-grade intraosseus sarcomas.

It is not clear which element of these protocols, the intraarterial drug, the radiation therapy, or the surgical excision, is responsible for the excellent local rate and high limb-salvage rate. It is possible that any one or all of them together contribute to the improved survival rate.

Microscopic extension beyond the visible and palpable tumor field is clearly the reason for local tumor recurrence in patients with extremity skeletal or soft-tissue sarcomas. Preoperative intraarterial Adriamycin and radiation produces a high percentage of tumor-cell necrosis. It is assumed that the microscopic peripheral extensions of the tumor are even more sensitive to the drug and radiation than are the large tumor masses that have been assayed for necrosis. The reduced local recurrence makes it probable that these assumptions are correct. Tumor-cell necrosis is difficult to quantitate, and there are geographic variations within these tumors in terms of which portion has been killed by the therapy. Nonetheless, it is amazing that there is marked evidence of tumor-cell necrosis within a relatively short period of time, from 1-2 weeks, in tumors that were previously very resistant to treatment.

Rosen et al. reported that systemic chemotherapy alone with cyclical Adriamycin or hydrous methotrexate could achieve a high incidence of tumor-cell necrosis; however, in approximately 50% of the patients this tumor-cell necrosis was less than 50% (18,19). We achieved an average tumor-cell necrosis of 90% in high-grade intraosseus osteosarcomas treated by additional radiation therapy.

The crucial question is whether the intraarterial drug route is superior to the intravenous route in this scheme (20,21). Although there are theoretic advantages to intraarterial Adriamycin, the practical facts are that this intraarterial administration is time-consuming for the patient, because it necessitates hospitalization and requires angiography, with its subsequent risks. Therefore, we feel it is very important to know whether the intraarterial route is superior. A randomized protocol is underway directly comparing intraarterial Adriamycin to intravenous Adriamycin, 1750 R radiation and surgical excision of extremity skeletal or soft-tissue sarcomas. Analyses of limb salvage, local tumor control, and assessment of tumor-cell necrosis will be compared to the present protocols.

Although amputation is necessary for some patients with extremity skeletal or soft-tissue sarcomas, it is clear from this study as well as from others that it is not necessary for most patients. Local tumor control is the goal of any primary tumor therapy, and it appears that multimodality therapy of chemotherapy, radiation, and surgery improves the local control rate for both skeletal and soft-tissue sarcomas. Although the long-term structural integrity of the salvaged extremity for both the skeletal and soft-tissue sarcoma patients remains in question, it certainly appears at a median follow-up of 5 years that the structural integrity has been maintained. The possibility of subsequent loosening of the metallic endoprosthesis remains a worrisome problem for patients with skeletal sarcomas. A longer follow-up will be necessary to determine how severe this problem may be.

REFERENCES

1. Martin R, Butler J: Soft tissue tumor — Surgical treatment and results. In: Tumors of Bone and Soft Tissue. Year Book Medical Publishers, Chicago, 1965, pp 333-347.
2. Shiu MH, Castro EB, Hajdu S: Surgical treatment of 297 soft-tissue sarcomas of the extremity. Ann Surg (182):597-602, 1975.
3. Gerner RE, Moore GE, Pickren JW: Soft tissue sarcomas. Ann Surg (181):803-808, 1975.
4. Rantakokko V, Ekfor TO: Sarcomas of the soft tissue in the extremities and limb girdles. Acta Chir Scand (145):385-394, 1979.

5. Markhede G, Angervoll L, Stenner B: A multivariant analysis of the prognosis after surgical treatment of malignant soft-tissue tumors. Cancer (49):1721-1733, 1981.
6. Enneking WF, Spanier SS, Malawer MM: The effect of the anatomic setting on the results of surgical procedures for soft-part sarcomas of the thigh. Cancer (47):1005-1022, 1981.
7. Lindberg R, Martin R, Ramsdahl M, Barkley T: Conservative surgery and postoperative radiotherapy in 300 adults with soft-tissue sarcoma. Cancer (47):2391-2397, 1981.
8. Lattuada A, Kenda R: Postoperative radiotherapy of soft-tissue sarcoma. Tumori (67):191, 1981.
9. Suit HD, Proppe KH, Mankin HJ, Wood WC: Radiation therapy and conservative surgery for sarcoma of soft-tissue. Prog Clin Cancer (8):311-318, 1982.
10. Gottlieb JA, Baker LH, O'Bryan RM, Sinkovics JG, Benjamin R: Adriamycin used alone and in combination for soft tissue and bony sarcomas. Cancer Chemother Rep (6):271-282, 1975.
11. Rudolph R, Stein R, Pattiuo R: Skin ulcers due to Adriamycin. Cancer (38):1087-1094, 1976.
12. Greco F, Brereton H, Kent H, Zimbler H, Merril J, Johnson R: Adriamycin and enhanced radiation reaction in normal esophagus and skin. Ann Int Med (85):294-298, 1976.
13. Haskell CM, Silverstein M, Rangel D, Hunt J, Sparks F, Morton D: Multimodality cancer therapy in man: A pilot study of adriamycin by arterial infusion. Cancer (33):1485-1490, 1974.
14. Eilber FR, Mirra JJ, Grant TT, Weisenburger T, Morton DL: Is amputation necessary for sarcomas? A 7-year experience with limb salvage. Ann Surg (192):431-437, 1980.
15. Eilber FR, Morton DL, Eckhardt J, Grant T, Weisenburger T: Limb salvage for skeletal and soft tissue sarcomas: Multidisciplinary preoperative therapy. Cancer, in press.
16. Tanigawa N, Kern DH, Hikasa Y, Morton DL: Rapid assay for evaluating the chemosensitivity of human tumors in soft agar culture. Cancer Res (42):2159-2164, 1982.
17. Kern DH, Bertelsen CA, Mann BD, Campbell MA, Morton DL, Cochran AJ: Clinical applications of the clonogenic assay. Ann Clin Lab Sci (13):10-15, 1983.
18. Rosen G, Nirenberg A: Chemotherapy for osteosarcoma: An investigative method, not a recipe. Cancer Treat Rep (66):1687-1697, 1982.
19. Rosen G, Capparos B, Huvos A, Kosloff C, Nirenberg A, Cacavio A, Marcove R, Lane J, Metha B: Preoperative chemotherapy for osteosarcoma: Selection of postoperative adjuvant chemotherapy based on the response of the primary tumor to chemotherapy. Cancer (49):1221-1230, 1982.
20. Kraybill W, Harrison M, Sasako T, Fletcher W: Regional intraarterial infusion of adriamycin in the treatment of cancer. Surg Gynecol & Obstet (144):335-338, 1977.
21. Didolkar M, Kanter P, Boffi R, Swartz H, Lopez R, Baez N: Comparison of regional versus systemic chemotherapy with adriamycin. Ann Surg (187):332-336, 1978.

PHASE I TRIALS AND PHARMACOKINETIC STUDIES OF INTRAPERITONEAL CISPLATIN, MELPHALAN, METHOTREXATE, AND CYTARABINE.

Stephen B. Howell, M.D., Craig E. Pfeifle, Pharm. D., Maurie Markman, M.D. Department of Medicine, Cancer Center, and General Clinical Research Center, University of California, San Diego, La Jolla, CA 92093.

ABSTRACT

Phase I and pharmacokinetic studies of the intraperitoneal administration of cisplatin, melphalan, methotrexate, and cytarabine have been completed at the UCSD Cancer Center. For all four agents, there is a very large pharmacologic advantage to administration via the intraperitoneal route. The mean ratio of total drug exposure for the peritoneal cavity to plasma was 12.4 (range 2.9-37.4) for cisplatin, 65 (range 17-176) for melphalan, 92 (range 7-303) for methotrexate, and 570 (range 320-1000) for cytarabine. The dose-limiting toxicity for all four agents was systemic rather than local, and the dose administered into the peritoneal cavity could be escalated to the point where the amount of drug leaking into the sytemic circulation provided a total drug exposure for the plasma equivalent to that which could be obtained with intravenous injection. In the case of cisplatin, concurrent systemic administration of sodium thiosulfate provided excellent protection for the kidneys and permitted escalation of the total intraperitoneal cisplatin dose to 270 mg/m^2. In the case of methotrexate and cytarabine, it was possible to maintain intraperitoneal concentrations well above the minimal cytotoxic level for ovarian carcinoma for a period of five days with acceptable systemic toxicity. The results indicate that these four drugs can be repeatedly administered into the peritoneal cavity and that this route of administration results in a very great pharmacologic advantage relative to systemic administration.

INTRODUCTION

Ovarian carcinoma characteristically remains confined to the peritoneal cavity for most of its natural history. Cells shed from the ovarian primary implant on the serosa of the abdominal organs and tend to grow on the surface rather than invade into the parenchyma. Although intravenously administered chemotherapeutic agents can reach that portion of the tumor that is fed by systemic capillaries, some components of the tumor reside at large diffusional distances away from the systemic circulation. On the basis of pharmacokinetic modelling, in 1978, Dedrick et al. (1) suggested that for some chemotherapeutic agents direct intraperitoneal instillation might be more advantageous than systemic administration. They pointed out that the peritoneal-to-plasma concentration ratio for drugs administered by intraperitoneal route should be greatest for drugs whose peritoneal clearance is extremely low, but whose systemic clearance is high. Stated another way, the ideal drug for intraperitoneal administration would be one that has a very difficult time getting out of the peritoneal cavity, but once it reaches the systemic circulation, is promptly removed so that there is minimal delivery of drug to bone marrow and gut.

Over the past five years, we have conducted a series of phase I and pharmacokinetic studies of three agents with established activity against ovarian carcinoma, cisplatin, melphalan, and methotrexate. In addition, based initially on the results of in vitro drug sensitivity testing, we have conducted a trial of intraperitoneal cytarabine and demonstrated its activity against ovarian carcinoma.

Intraperitoneal Cisplatin with Systemic Thiosulfate Protection

In this study (2,3), cisplatin was administered intraperitoneally in 2 liters of normal saline and allowed to dwell in the abdomen for four hours. Patients were hydrated with normal saline intravenously for 12 hours before treatment and were given intravenous mannitol for 6 hours after intraperitoneal drug instillation. When 90 mg/m^2 of cisplatin was instilled, the mean peak serum creatinine increase during the three weeks after treatment was 55%. When sodium thiosulfate 2 g/m^2 per hour for 12 hours was started concurrently with the intraperitoneal cisplatin instillation, there was complete protection against nephrotoxicity (Figure 1), but, importantly, it was then possible to escalate the dose of cisplatin to 270 mg/m^2 without producing nephrotoxicity. Even 270 mg/m^2 was not a maximum tolerated dose. Vomiting was universal, and although cisplatin regularly produced a transient drop in leukocyte and platelet counts, even at the 270 mg/m^2 dose level, the mean white count nadir was only 3,800/mm^3, and the platelet nadir was 113,000/mm^3.

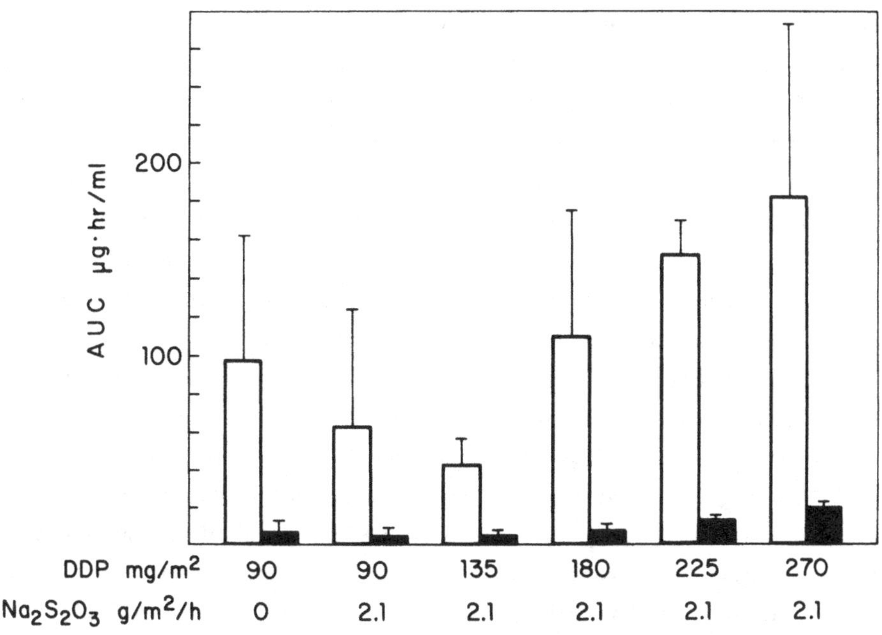

Figure 1

Figure 1: The mean area under the curve for free reactive cisplatin in peritoneal dialysate (open bars) and plasma (closed bars) as a function of cisplatin and sodium thiosulfate doses. Vertical lines indicate standard deviations.

Only one of the 17 patients treated developed any evidence of chemical peritonitis, and subsequent cycles of intraperitoneal cisplatin therapy at escalated doses were not associated with any local toxicity in this patient. There was no gross or histologic evidence of damage to the serosa surfaces within the peritoneal cavity after up to three courses of treatment.

When total active cisplatin (that fraction not yet neutralized by sodium thiosulfate) was measured by high pressure liquid chromatography, total drug exposure for the peritoneal cavity was found to be an average of 12-fold greater than that for the plasma. At a dose of 90 mg/m^2 without sodium thiosulfate, exposure for the plasma was approximately half of that which would have been achieved by an intravenous infusion of 100 mg/m^2 of cisplatin; at 270 mg/m^2 of cisplatin intraperitoneally, the plasma drug exposure was approximately twice that which would have been produced by a maximum tolerated dose of cisplatin given intravenously (2,3). Thus, the combination of intraperitoneal cisplatin and intravenous sodium thiosulfate results in the unique situation where not only does the peritoneal cavity receive an extremely high total drug exposure, but the amount of drug delivered to the systemic circuit is also approximately twice that which could be delivered by a maximum tolerated intravenous dose of cisplatin without sodium thiosulfate.

This suggests that sodium thiosulfate is not neutralizing very much platinum in the plasma. This has been confirmed in subsequent studies of intravenously administered cisplatin with intravenous sodium thiosulfate (4,5). In addition, we have demonstrated that sodium thiosulfate is concentrated approximately 25-fold in the urine (6). Our current hypothesis is that neutralization of cisplatin in the kidney is excellent, but it is not very good in the rest of the body. This is corroborated by the fact that sodium thiosulfate does not appear to protect against nausea and vomiting, myelosuppression, or neurotoxicity.

Three of the 12 evaluable patients on this study demonstrated responses despite the fact that they all had very advanced disease.

Intraperitoneal Chemotherapy with Melphalan

Nineteen patients were treated with intraperitoneal instillations of escalating doses of melphalan in 2 liters of fluid using a 4-hour dwell time (7). The dose was escalated from 30-90 mg/m^2. The dose-limiting toxicity was reached at 70 mg/m^2 and was myelosuppression rather than local peritoneal toxicity. At this dose, the mean white blood count nadir was 2,000/mm^3, and the mean platelet nadir was 69,000/mm^3.

No patient to date has developed clinical symptoms or signs of peritonitis. There was no increase in the number of inflammatory cells in the peritoneal fluid with serial courses of treatment and no suggestion of progressive sclerosis of the cavity. The median number of courses administered was 2. Five patients underwent laparotomy or autopsy within 4 weeks of receiving intraperitoneal melphalan, and none had gross or microscopic evidence of serosal changes that could be attributed to treatment. However, in patients receiving a large number of courses, pseudomembrane formation over the small intestine was observed. Intraperitoneal melphalan did not produce any short term abnormalities of hepatic function.

The mean ratio of peak peritoneal concentration to peak plasma concentration was 93; the minimun ratio in any patient was 24, and the maximum ratio was 291. The ratio of total drug exposure for the peritoneal cavity to that for the plasma averaged 65, with a range of from 17 to 176. Thus, at all dose levels, intraperitoneal administration of melphalan resulted in a much greater total drug exposure for the peritoneal cavity than for plasma. One of 14 evaluable ovarian carcinoma patients had a complete response lasting 12+ months.

This study showed that melphalan could be administered by the intraperitoneal route with safety and demonstrated that there is a tremendous pharmacologic advantage for the intraperitoneal, as opposed to the intravenous or oral, administration of melphalan. The maximum tolerated intraperitoneal dose is approximately 3-fold larger than the maximum tolerated intravenous dose. Thus, if any part of the tumor is accessible to intraperitoneally instilled drug, there is no rationale from a pharmacologic point of view for the use of intravenous or oral routes, rather than the intraperitoneal route,for the administration of melphalan.

TABLE 1: The Hematologic Toxicity of Melphalan Administered by the Intraperitoneal Route.

Melphalan Dose mg/m^2	No. Patients	No. Courses	10^{-3} x WBC (cells/mm^3)		10^{-3} x Platelets (cells/mm^3)	
			Pretreatment Mean*(range)	Nadir Mean*(range)	Pretreatment Mean*(range)	Nadir Mean*(range)
30	4	4	4.4(2.3-6.5)	3.5(2.9-5.1)	335(221-607)	280(178-578)
40	4	9	5.0(3.5-6.4)	3.8(3.0-5.4)	198(100-578)	131(42-579)
50	5	7	4.0(2.9-5.6)	2.8(1.0-5.5)	243(188-339)	176(128-381)
60	7	8	4.6(3.8-6.6)	2.8(0.6-5.9)	289(178-441)	133(25-334)
70	8	12	5.1(3.0-13.0)	2.0(0.2-7.2)	283(181-707)	69(9-395)
80	2	2	4.3(3.1-6.1)	1.0(0.2-4.9)	340(313-371)	44(10-192)
90	1	1	5.2	4.3	266	231

*Geometric mean

TABLE 2. The Pharmacokinetics of Melphalan Administered by the Intraperitoneal Route.

		Peritoneal				Plasma		Ratio*	
Dose mg/m^2	No. Courses Evaluable	Peak Concentration ug/ml mean (S.D.)	Halflife hrs mean (S.D.)	AUC_{ip} ug·hr/ml mean (S.D.)	Clearance $L/hr/m^2$ mean (S.D.)	Peak Concentration ug/ml mean (S.D.)	AUC_{pl} ug·hr/ml mean (S.D.)	Peak Concentration mean (S.D.)	AUC mean (S.D.)
30	4	5.5 (2.5)	1.0 (0.4)	10.0 (5.5)	0.76 (0.11)	0.094 (0.005)	0.20 (0.02)	49 (22)	49 (24)
40	7	21.5 (8.9)	1.1 (0.2)	39.1 (12.0)	0.80 (0.21)	0.267 (0.166)	0.72 (0.06)	101 (48)	91 (64)
50	4	32.4 (10.6)	1.1 (0.4)	55.0 (12.8)	0.96 (0.04)	0.333 (0.126)	0.96 (0.40)	100 (23)	60 (10)
60	6	27.1 (5.2)	1.0 (0.2)	52.1 (37.9)	0.84 (0.21)	0.403 (0.250)	1.42 (0.92)	80 (48)	46 (36)
70	4	19.4 (16.7)	0.8 (0.4)	38.9 (23.7)	0.99 (0.35)	0.306 (0.289)	0.91 (0.85)	110 (114)	82 (73)
80	1	16.1	1.4	26.6	0.65	0.445	1.86	36	14

*Peritoneal/plasma

Intraperitoneal Methotrexate with Systemic Leucovorin Protection

Methotrexate is a cell cycle stage-specific drug, and its toxicity is a function not only of its concentration, but also of the duration of exposure. For slow-growing tumors such as ovarian carcinoma, the rational way to use this drug would be to keep it in contact with the tumor for very long periods of time. We conducted a phase I trial of the constant intraperitoneal infusion of methotrexate with concurrent administration of just enough leucovorin into the systemic circulation to neutralize the methotrexate reaching the plasma (8). Eighteen patients with malignant effusions were treated with intraperitoneal infusions of 30 mg/m^2 of methotrexate per day. Leucovorin, 15 mg/m^2 loading dose and 10 mg/m^2 maintenance dose, was injected intravenously every 4 hours for the duration of the methotrexate infusion and then every 6 hours until the serum methotrexate levels were less than 50 nM. It was demonstrated by in vitro studies of human bone marrow that, as long as the peritoneal concentrations of methotrexate were 10-fold greater than the plasma concentration, even if the leucovorin diffused into the peritoneal cavity, it would not be expected to interfere with the antitumor activity of methotrexate in the cavity. Figure 2 demonstrates that steady state was reached after 12 hours of intraperitoneal infusion, and the mean steady-state peritoneal to plasma methotrexate concentration ratio was 92.

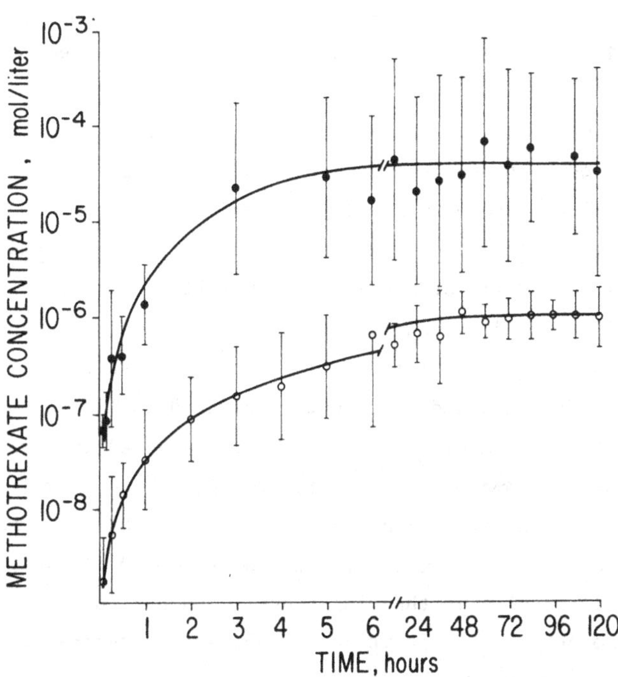

Figure 2

Figure 2: Geometric mean MTX concentration in the serum (O) and effusions (O) of four patients with malignant ascites as a function of time after the start of intraperitoneal MTX infusion. Mean ± SD.

The duration of total peritoneal infusion of methotrexate was incrementally increased from 1-5 days, and even at 5 days changes in white blood count and platelet count, which were the major form of toxicity, were of moderate degree. Serial cytokinetic analysis of the bone marrow demonstrated no evidence of methotrexate effect.

Three of 8 patients with far advanced disease demonstrated responses lasting 13, 10, and 20+ months.

The major significance of this study was that it demonstrated, really for the first time, that it is possible to use a cell cycle stage specific antimetabolite in a rational way against ovarian carcinoma. Methotrexate concentrations averaged 24 uM in the peritoneal cavity, well above the minimal cytotoxic level for ovarian carcinoma.

Intraperitoneal Cytarabine Chemotherapy in Ovarian Carcinoma

Although ara-C is not known to be an active drug against ovarian carcinoma, in vitro drug sensitivity testing using the Hamburger-Salmon technique demonstrated activity of this drug against five of nine patients with far advanced ovarian carcinoma (9). The pharmacokinetics of intraperitoneally administered ara-C were studied in three patients with ovarian carcinoma. When the drug was instilled in 2 liters of normal saline at concentrations of 10, 100, and 1,000 um, the peritoneal kinetics were first order with half-lives of 70-120 minutes. Plasma ara-C was not detected in the plasma until the peritoneal concentration was raised to 100 uM; the peritoneal-to-plasma concentration ratio for ara-C approximated 1,000.

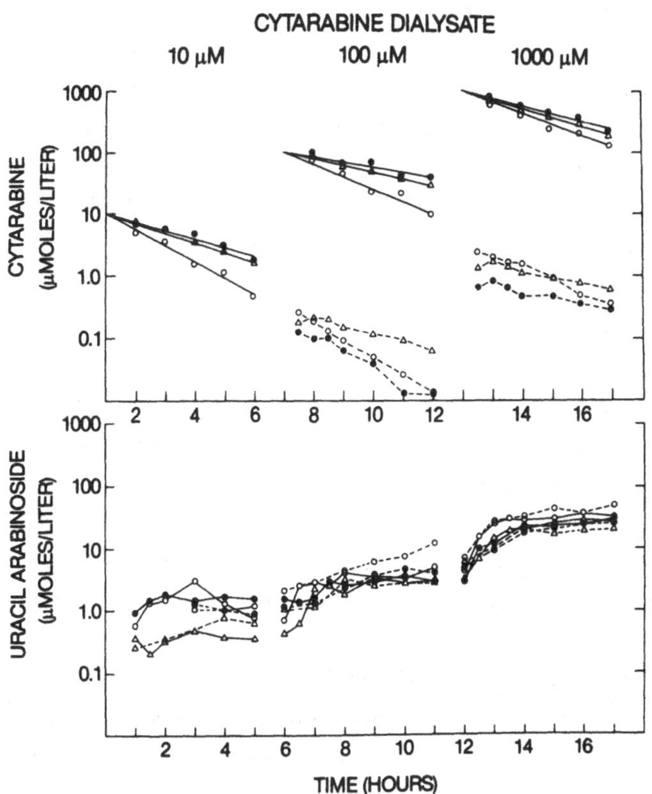

Figure 3

Figure 3: Plasma and peritoneal cytarabine (upper panel) and uracil arabinoside (lower panel) concentrations found during consecutive peritoneal dialysate exchanges of 10, 100, and 1000 uM cytarabine in three patients with advanced ovarian carcinoma.

These results confirm the predictions made on the basis of pharmacokinetic modelling by Dedrick et al. (1).

Encouraged by the pharmacokinetic results, 10 patients with advanced ovarian carcinoma were treated with a constant peritoneal dialysis of 60 uM ara-C exchanged every 6 hours for a total of five days. This treatment produced only mild nausea and mild myelosuppression. The entrance criteria required a white blood count of greater than 3,000/mm^3 and a platelet count of greater than 100,000/mm^3. The mean nadir white blood count following treatment was 3,700/mm^3, and only one of 25 cycles was associated with a platelet count of less than 75,000/mm^3.

Two of the 10 evaluable patients had complete responses, and these have now lasted 14+ and 15+ months since the end of treatment.

Like the situation with methotrexate, this study demonstrated that ara-C could be maintained at cytotoxic concentrations in the intraperitoneal cavity for up to 5 days and established that this form of treatment was capable of producing complete remissions in patients with ovarian carcinoma who had failed primary therapy.

SUMMARY

For all four of the drugs studied in this series of phase I and pharmacokinetic investigations, the intraperitoneal route of administration offers a tremendous pharmacologic advantage. There was clearly no toxicity to the major intra-abdominal organs. There was also little evidence of damage to the peritoneal surfaces. However, it should be noted that only a few of these patients received multiple courses of therapy. Adhesions, fibrosis, and sclerosis of the peritoneal cavity may become a problem with multiple courses of treatment. In the case of cisplatin, the combination of this agent with sodium thiosulfate permitted a doubling of the amount of active cisplatin reaching the systemic circulation since it provided excellent renal protection. The studies with methotrexate and ara-C demonstrated that the intraperitoneal route not only permits extremely high concentrations to be achieved at the surfaces of tumor but also permits very long duration of exposure without undue systemic toxicity. It now remains to be demonstrated whether the tremendous pharmacologic advantage demonstrated in these studies can be translated into improved therapy for patients with advanced tumors confined to the peritoneal cavity.

REFERENCES

1. Dedrick, R.L., Myers, C.E., Bungay, P.M., and DeVita, V.T. Jr. Pharmacokinetic rationale for peritoneal drug administration in the treatment of ovarian cancer. Cancer Treatment Reports 62:1-9, 1978.
2. Howell, S.B., Pfeifle, C.E., Wung, W.E., Olshen, R.A., Lucas, W.E., Yon, J.L., and Green, M. Intraperitoneal Cisplatin with Systemic Thiosulfate Protection. Annals of Internal Medicine 97:845-851, 1982.
3. Howell, S.B., Pfeifle, C.E., Wung, W.E., Olshen, R.A. Intraperitoneal cisplatin with systemic thiosulfate protection. Cancer Research 43:1426-1431, 1983.
4. Campbell, T.N., Howell, S.B., Pfeifle, C.E., Wung, W.E., Bookstein, J. Pharmacokinetics of intra-arterial cisplatin in man. Cancer Research, in press, 1984.
5. Woliver, T., Felthouse, R., Markman, M., Pfeifle, C.E., Howell, S.B. Phase I trial of intravenous cisplatin (DDP) with sodium thiosulfate protection. Proc. Am. Assoc. Cancer Res. 24:132, 1983.
6. Shea, M., Koziol, J.A., Howell, S.B. Human pharmacokinetics of sodium thiosulfate, a neutralizing agent for cisplatin. Clinical Pharmacol. and Therap., in press, 1983.
7. Pfeifle, C.E., Howell, S.B., Olshen, R.A. Intraperitoneal (I.P.) melphalan (L-PAM): a phase I study. Am. Soc. Clin. Pharmacol. Therap. 33:223, 1983.
8. Howell, S.B., Chu, B.C.F., Wung, W., Metha, B., Mendelsohn, J. Long duration intracavitary infusion of methotrexate with systemic leucovorin protection in patients with malignant effusions. J. Clin. Invest. 67:1167-1170, 1981.
9. King, M.E., Smith, A., Young, B., and Howell, S.B. Modulation of cytarabine uptake and toxicity by dipyridamole. Cancer Treatment Reports, in press, 1984.

Supported in part by grants CA 23100 and CA 35309 from the National Institutes of Health, by grant RR-008827 from the National Institutes of Health, Division of Research Resources, and by a grant from the Dr. Louis Sklarow Memorial Fund. This work was conducted in part by the Clayton Foundation for Cancer Research - California Division. Dr. Howell is a Clayton Foundation Investigator.

A PHASE I TRIAL OF INTRACAVITARY DOXORUBICIN (ADRIAMYCIN) ALTERNATING WITH CISPLATIN

KAREN ANTMAN, ROBERT OSTEEN, DIANE MONTELLA

INTRODUCTION

A substantial pharmacologic advantage might be gained by delivering chemotherapy directly into the peritoneum or pleura for tumors confined to these serous cavities. Peak drug levels in ascites after intraperitoneal administration range from 30 to 474 times that achieved in plasma after intravenous (IV) dosage. (Table 1) If a drug has a high level of hepatic extraction, the plasma concentration after intracavitary (IC) administration of a given dose may be substantially lower than that after IV administration. Thus, the systemic toxicity for IC administration may also be considerably less than that for the same dose of the drug given IV. Phase I and pharmacokinetic studies have been published for IC administration of doxorubicin (Adriamycin), 5 flourouracil, methotrexate, and cisplatin (DDP) as single agents. (1-12) In addition, bleomycin and doxorubicin have been administered IC in an effort to control effusions, although no pharmacology studies were performed. (9,13,14) (Table 1)

Table 1. Intracavitary (IC) chemotherapy.

Drug	Institute	Pts.	Max. Dose /course	Peak Levels IC Plasma	Dose Limiting Toxicity	$T_{1/2}$(hr)	%Absorbed /x hrs	Responses
Doxorubicin	NCI(1-3)	10	60 mg	474	Abd. Pain*	1.6	85/4	3/10
5-Fluorouracil	NCI(4)	10	9 g	298	Myelosup.**	1.6	82/4	2/8
Methotrexate with rescue	NCI(5-6)	5	500 uMx48 hr	36	Abd. Pain	NT	70/5	0/5
Cisplatin	UCSD(7)	17	270 mg/m^2	33	N/V***	0.9		3/12
Cisplatin	MSKCC(8)	6	60 mg/m^2	30	None			1/6
Bleomycin	Albany(9)	38	240 mg/m^2		Fever, rash			"63%"

*Abdominal Pain
**Myelosuppression
***Nausea/Vomiting

NCI: National Cancer Institute
USCD: University of California at San Diego
MSKCC: Memorial Sloan Kettering Cancer Center

METHODS

Eligibility requirements included histologically proven malignancy, and either disease confined to the pleura or peritoneum, or major morbidity resulting from tumor in these locations. Measurable disease was not required. When appropriate and feasible, gross tumor was surgically removed prior to IC therapy. Patients must have refused, failed, or been ineligible for any curative or conventional palliative treatment. Failure to respond to IV administration of doxorubicin or cisplatin did not render a patient ineligible.

IC chemotherapy was first administered at least four weeks after prior chemotherapy or radiation therapy. Chemotherapy was delayed at least one week after surgical placement of a Tenckhoff or Port-a-Cath Catheter (Pharmacia Nu-Tech, Piscataway, New Jersey).

To insure relatively safe drug delivery, the following parameters were required prior to entry:

White Cell Count	>3,500/ul
Platelet Count	>100,000/ul
Hemoglobin	>10 mg/dl
BUN	<25 mg/dl
Creatinine	<1.5 mg/dl*
Bilirubin	<1.5 mg/dl

*Creatinine Clearance: ≥55 ml/minute for any course involving platinum.

All patients entering the study were informed of the investigational nature of the treatment as well as the therapeutic results and toxicity which might be reasonably anticipated. No concurrent medical or psychiatric illness which would have prevented informed consent or limited intensive treatment was allowed, including uncontrolled infection or severe cardiovascular disease, such as myocardial infarction in the last six months or congestive heart failure requiring digoxin.

Method of Drug Administration

Drug was diluted in 1-2 liters of peritoneal dialysate and injected through a semi-permanently implanted Tenckhoff or Port-a-Cath delivery system. However, for patients with large collections of ascites or for pleural effusions, the drug was diluted into 250 ml of normal saline and administered through a temporary percutaneously placed polyethylene catheter.

<u>Chemotherapy</u>

Patients initially received two escalating doses of doxorubicin. If doxorubicin was well tolerated, then cisplatin (DDP) was administered on day 14 following doxorubicin. Drugs were alternated with doxorubicin day 1, DDP day 14, on a 21-day cycle. This interval was chosen to allow for resolution of any peritonitis prior to DDP administration. Doses were escalated both within and between patients, with three administrations per level if no significant toxicity resulted. Five administrations per patient level were given when a significant but reversible toxicity was observed.

Chemical peritonitis or pleuritis was anticipated as the dose - limiting toxicity for single-agent IC doxorubicin. The dose at which the patient developed 1+ abdominal or chest discomfort was documented. (Table 2) That same dose was then given at the time of the next scheduled doxorubicin treatment, this time with prednisone 20 mg TID for three days. The dose of doxorubicin was then escalated again until the development of 1+ abdominal or chest discomfort occurred on steroids.

TABLE 2. Chemical peritonitis or pleuritis.

1+ : <24 hours of mild abdominal discomfort.
2+ : 1-3 days of abdominal or chest discomfort requiring analgesics.
3+ : 3-10 days of abdominal or chest pain requiring codeine analgesics.

Cisplatin was held if the creatinine clearance fell below 55 ml/minute. Fifty percent of the dose of chemotherapy was not given if, on the day of scheduled treatment, the white blood count was between 2,000-3,000/ul, or platelets between 50,000-70,000/ul.

<u>Response Criteria</u>:

Standard criteria were used for responses in patients with measurable disease. Pleural or peritoneal effusions were not considered measurable but were evaluable for assessing palliation.

<u>Complete response</u>: disappearance of all measurable disease as well as tumor-associated signs, symptoms and biochemical changes for four weeks or more, during which no new lesions appeared and no existing lesions enlarged.

A partial response: a reduction of $\geq$4 weeks duration of 50% in the sum of the products of the perpendicular diameters of all measurable lesions, with the appearance of no new lesions, nor enlargement of existing lesions.

Stable disease: a <50% reduction or <25% increase of $\geq$8 weeks duration in the sum of the products of two perpendicular diameters of all measured lesions, and the appearance of no new lesions.

Objective progressions or relapse: an increase in the product of two perpendicular diameters of any measured lesion by >25% over the size present at entry on study or the appearance of any new lesions.

The maximum tolerated dose: the dose of drug that, at the schedule tested, produces predictable and reversible toxicity: either myelosuppression with a WBC nadir between 1,000 and 2,000/ul and platelets between 40-80,000/ul, or any other toxicity which is either transiently incapacitating or interferes with the patient's well being and general activities.

RESULTS

Eighteen patients were entered. (Table 3) The peritoneal cavity was treated in 16, the pleural cavity in three. (One patient had both peritoneal and right pleural cavities treated sequentially.) Drug was instilled at the time of repeated thoracentesis or paracentesis via a temporary percutaneously placed polyethylene catheter in seven patients with large effusions. A Tenckhoff catheter drug delivery system was used in seven patients, and a Port-a-Cath system in four more recently treated patients.

A total of 91 courses were delivered (59 doxorubicin and 32 cisplatin). (Table 4) Patients received a range of 1-20 (median 3) treatments. Three patients had received no prior chemotherapy, 10 had received one prior regimen, and five patients had received two or more. Five had had radiotherapy. Two complete and three partial remissions as well as disease progression in two patients had resulted from prior regimens. The remainder had inevaluable disease at the time of prior chemotherapy.

Table 3. Patient summaries arranged by number of courses delivered.

Age	Sex	Histology	# OF COURSES #C	ADR	DDP	HIGHEST DOSE ADR mg	DDP/m^2	BEST RESPONSE		TOXICITY ADR	DDP	Miscellaneous
50	F	Ovary	1+		1		70	I	Too early.			
50	F	Ovary	1		1		100	I	Died: CVA after 1 wk.			
70	F	Mesothelioma	1	1		40		SD	No change in effusion.			
61	F	Mesothelioma	1	1		40		SD	No change in effusion.			
68	F	Gastric	1	1		25		SD	No change in effusion.			
47	F	Breast	2	1	1	54	70	R	No abd tumor at autopsy.	3+ peritonitis	Ileus, Creat 3.0	
65	F	Fallopian Tube	2	2		50		SD	No change in effusion.			
43	M	Renal	2	2		45		SD	No change in effusion.	Nausea x3 days		
60	M	Biliary	3	3		40		SD	No change in effusion.	Abd pain		
27	M	Mesothelioma	3+	1	2	35	90	SD	No progression x2 mo.	Localized pain	Ileus, creat 1.3, WBC 1.9, Plts 44,000	Difficulty delivering diluent
51	M	Mesothelioma	3+	1	2	20	90	SD	No progression x1 mo.		Hiccoughs	Catheter clotted; replaced
54	M	Liposarcoma	4	4		45		DP	Developed small bowel obstruction.			Catheter leak; replaced
54	F	Fallopian Tube	8	5	3	40	35	SD	Weight gain.	3+ peritonitis	Pain with infusion due to adhesions	Difficulty delivering diluent
54	F	Ovary	8	3	5	50	90	R	Ascites resolved, pl effusion x 6 mo.			
34	F	Mesothelioma	9	5	3	45	75	R	Disappearance of 7 mm lesions.			
74	M	Mesothelioma	9+	6	3	60	120	SD	No progression x5 mo.		WBC 2.0, Plts 77,000	S. Aureus peritonitis
41	M	Mesothelioma	10	3	7	50	90	SD	No progression x13 mo.			
52	M	Mesothelioma	20	18	2	90	75	R	Decreased ascites, wt. gain x16 mo.	Extravasation	Ileus, dehydration	Catheter Leak

I: Inevaluable
R: Response

SD: Stable disease
DP: Disease progression

abd: abdominal

Table 4. Number of courses delivered at each dose level.

Dose level*	Doxorubicin	Cisplatin
<25	3	2
30	11	3
40	13	3
45	6	2
50	9	3
60	3	0
70	2	7
80	6	3
90	4	7
100	0	1
120	0	1
	59	32

*Doxorubicin in mg total dose, cisplatin in mg/m^2.

Toxicity

Doxorubicin: Doxorubicin toxicity was chiefly mild to moderate abdominal pain beginning 20-24 hours after treatment and continuing for one to three days. Dialysate could not be delivered freely (presumably because of adhesions) in two patients who developed prolonged localized pain after delivery of doxorubicin doses generally well tolerated by other patients. One patient given a first dose of 54 mg had severe abdominal pain and was unable to eat for seven days. However, a total of eight courses were delivered in other patients at 50 mg total dose, and 13 courses at higher doxorubicin dosages were given with mild to moderate abdominal pain observed.

Another patient tolerated repeated doxorubicin doses of up to 90 mg per dose but required prednisone 20 mg TID to control pain. He received a total dose of doxorubicin of 1090 mg/m^2 (450 mg/m^2 IV, then 640 mg/m^2 IP) with no evidence of cardiotoxicity (clinically or at autopsy).

Extravasation of doxorubicin into the abdominal wall occurred during delivery of a single course via a 16-guage paracentesis catheter. A 2-3 cm ellipse of skin, muscle and fascia around the extravasation was excised at the time of surgical placement of a Tenckhoff catheter.

Even after 90 mg doses, there was no evident myelosuppression, although red urine and mild nausea were occasionally observed. There was no alopecia.

Seventeen patients received IC doxorubicin. Eight had only one IC dose of doxorubicin and therefore did not receive prednisione.

Prednisone was contraindicated in two others because of hypertension or diabetes. Of the seven remaining patients, peritonitis was eliminated in four patients with 1-2+ discomfort. (Table 5) One patient routinely required six days of prednisone after 70-90 mg doses of IC doxorubicin. Delivery of the drug was difficult in two patients with presumed adhesions. Both developed localized abdominal pain lasting up to a week. One had no pain while on steroids, developing pain on day four when the steroids were discontinued, with relief again when given an additional course of three days of prednisone. The second patient required narcotics in spite of prednisone.

Table 5. IC Chemotherapy: prednisone for ADR peritonitis.

Dose: 20 mg TID x 3 days

17 patients received IC Doxorubicin
- 10 Inevaluable:
  - One dose only 8
  - Diabetic, hypertensive 2
- 7 Evaluable:
  - <u>1-2+ Toxicity</u>: Eliminated in all 4 patients.
    Most tolerated ~10 mg more drug.
  - <u>3+ Toxicity</u>: 2 with adhesions & localized pain.
    - 1 incomplete relief.
    - 1 complete relief, but relapsed day 4. (pred x3 more days with relief).

    1 required x6 days/course for 90 mg.

<u>Cisplatin</u>: Cisplatin regularly caused moderate to severe nausea and vomiting. Two to three days of ileus and dehydration were observed after three courses delivered at 50, 70, and 90 mg/m^2. The creatinine of the second patient rose from 0.9 to 3.0, subsequently falling slowly to 1.0. This patient had received cisplatin shortly after recovery from severe doxorubicin-induced chemical peritonitis (and thus may have had more rapid cisplatin uptake or may have been more dehydrated than most patients). The creatinine in the third patient rose from 1.0 to 1.3 mg/dl on day 3 but returned promptly to 0.9 mg/dl with hydration.

Only three patients had white blood count nadirs between 1,900/ul and 3,000/ul after cisplatin. Two had received prior pelvic radiation, and one prior mitomycin C. Platelet nadirs in these patients were between 40,000/ul and 77,000/ul. Marrow recovery was slow (up to six weeks).

Miscellaneous Complications

Two infections were treated. *Staph. aureaus* peritonitis in one patient responded to two weeks of IV oxacillin (without removal of the Tenckhoff catheter). Gram stain of ascites from the second patient revealed at least four organisms, suggesting bowel perforation rather than an infected Tenckhoff as the cause, a finding confirmed at laparotomy. Post-mortem examination revealed a cytomegalic infection with the organisms obstructing capillaries in the intestinal wall. Multiple perforations of the ischemic intestinal wall were identified.

Responses

Most patients had ascites or pleural effusions, but, as in many other phase I studies, measurable disease was not required. In addition, initial patients on the study received doses which would be unlikely to be therapeutic. Of the total of 18 patients (Table 3), two are totally inevaluable. (One has just had the first treatment; one died of a stroke one week after receiving 100 mg/m^2 of intraperitoneal cisplatin.)

Of patients with evaluable but unmeasurable disease, six with recurrent ascites or effusion discontinued IC therapy after one to three doxorubicin treatments at doses of 25-50 mg. One patient who seemed to have a somewhat better performance status after IC therapy refused further treatment. Four patients with nodules of malignant mesothelioma scattered throughout the abdomen at the time of insertion of a semi-permanent catheter (but no measurable disease by ultrasonagram or CAT scan) have had no documented disease progression for 1, 2, 5, and 13 months.

A 50-year-old male with malignant mesothelioma, who had required weekly evacuation of four to six liters of ascites, obtained significant relief of his abdominal distention over the 18 months of treatment (20 courses). He gained weight and was able to return to work for approximately one year. At autopsy, tumor involved the retroperitoneum and had immobilized the bowel loops. However, the anterior surface of the bowel was grossly free of tumor. This may represent either an unusual pattern of tumor growth or a response.

A 54-year-old woman with ovarian cancer presented with ascites, having failed IV cyclophosphamide, doxorubicin, and cisplatin. Two courses of doxorubicin intraperitoneally did not substantially change production of four to six liters of ascites each week. After four cycles of cisplatin at doses of 50 to 90 mg/m^2/course, there was no longer enough ascites present to allow safe needle entry for drug delivery. She has had no recurrent ascites for six months without treatment. A pleural effusion which contained neoplastic cells later developed but did not recur after one intrapleural instillation of 75 mg/m^2 of cisplatin.

Of the three patients with measurable disease, a 35-year-old woman with mesothelioma, who initially had multiple 0.7 cm nodules throughout the abdominal cavity, had a second-look laparotamy at the time the Tenckhoff catheter was removed. Several nodules remained in an area of an adhesion, but all other tumor had regressed completely. These nodules were resected, and the patient then received post-operative whole abdominal radiotherapy. She remains clinically well 18 months after diagnosis. A second patient had rare malignant cells on cytocentrifuge. After two treatments with considerable toxicity, malignant cells were no longer observed. No peritoneal tumor was observed at autopsy. A third patient with liposarcoma clearly progressed, developing small bowel obstruction while receiving intracavitary doxorubicin.

DISCUSSION

Total doses of 35 mg of doxorubicin alternating with 90 mg/m^2 of cisplatin may be safely administered intraperitoneally in patients who are able to tolerate at least 1-2 liters of diluent. Doxorubicin may then be escalated at 5 mg increments in individual patients. Lower doses should be considered if starting one to two weeks after major surgical resections. Severe localized pain will result if the drug is delivered into a small cavity which has been segregated from the free peritoneal cavity by adhesions. Omentectomy and postoperative intraperitoneal instillation of manitol may limit adhesions. Patients appeared to tolerate about a 10 mg higher dose of intracavitary doxorubicin if prednisone 20 mg TID was administered by mouth for 3 days, beginning with each treatment course. Insufficient numbers of patients were treated to reliably evaluate this effect. The toxicity of cisplatin appeared to be enhanced by recent doxorubicin-induced chemical peritonitis. Of three patients developing late (day 3-5) ileus and subsequent dehydration after cisplatin, two developed a transient elevation in creatinine. No other patients had renal toxicity. Hair loss was conspicuously absent. Myelosuppression was not observed after doxorubicin therapy, but WBC nadirs as low as 1,900/ul were observed after cisplatin therapy in two patients with prior pelvic irradiation and in one with prior mitomycin C.

Intracavitary chemotherapy can be clearly palliative in patients with recurrent ascites. In patients with multiple nodules of less than 1 cm in size, IC combination chemotherapy may result in a substantial response if adhesions protecting these lesions can be prevented.

REFERENCES

1. Ozols RF, Young RC, Speyer JL, Sugarbaker PH, Greene R, Jenkins J, Myers CE: Phase I and pharmacological studies of Adriamycin administered intraperitoneally to patients with ovarian cancer. Cancer Res (42): 4265-4269, 1982.

2. Ozols RF, Willson JKV, Grotzinger KR, Young RC: Cloning of human ovarian cancer cells in soft agar from malignant effusions and peritoneal washings. Cancer Res (40): 2743-2747, 1980.

3. Ozols RF, Willson JKV, Weltz MD, Grotzinger KR, Myers CE, Young RC: Inhibition of human ovarian cancer colony formation by Adriamycin and its major metabolites. Cancer Res (40): 4109-4112, 1980.

4. Speyer JL, Collins JM, Dedric RL, Brennan MF, Londer H, DeVita VT, Myers CE: Phase I and pharmacological studies of 5-Fluorouracil administered intraperitoneally. Cancer Res (40): 567-572, 1980.

5. Jones RB, Myers CE, Guarino AM, Dedrick RL, Hubbard SM, DeVita VT: High-volume intraperitoneal chemotherapy ("belly bath") for ovarian cancer. Cancer Chemother Pharmacol (1): 1161-1166, 1978.

6. Jones RB, Collins JM, Myers CE, Brooks AE, Hubbard SM, Ballow JW, Brennan MF, Dedrick RJ, DeVita VT: High-volume intraperitoneal chemotherapy with methotrexate in patients with cancer. Cancer Res (41): 55-59, 1981.

7. Howell SB, Pfeifle CE, Wung WE, Olshen RA, Lucas WE, Yon JL, Green M: Intraperitoneal Cisplatin with systemic thiosulphate protection. Ann Intern Med (97): 845-851, 1982.

8. Casper ES, Kelsen DP, Alcock NW, Lewis JL Jr: Pharmacokinetic study of intraperitoneal (IP) Cisplatin (CP) in patients with malignant ascites. Proc ASCO (1): 22(C-87), 1982.

9. Paladine WP, Cunningham TJ, Sponzo R. Donovan M, Olson K, Horton J: Intracavitary bleomycin in the management of malignant effusions. Cancer (38): 1903-1908, 1976.

10. Dedrick RL, Myers CL, Bungay PM, DeVita VT Jr: Pharmokinetic rationale for peritoneal drug administration in the treatment of ovarian cancer. Cancer Treat Rep (62): 1-11, 1978.

11. Ozols RF, Looker GY, Doroshow JH, Grotzinger KR, Myers CE, Young RC: Pharmacokinetics of Adriamycin and tissue penetration in murine ovarian cancer. Cancer Res (39): 3209-3214, 1979.

12. Roboz J, Chahinian AP, Tosk J, Holland JF: Transport of doxorubicin from peritoneal fluid to plasma in malignant mesothelioma. Proc AACR (22): 229(#906), 1981.

13. Kefford Rf, Woods RL, Fox RM, Tattersall MHN: Intracavitary Adriamycin, nitrogen mustard and tetracycline in the control of malignant effusions. Med J Australia (2): 447-448, 1980.

14. Tattersall MHN, Fox RM, Newlands ES, Woods RL: Intracavitary doxorubicin in malignant effusions. Lancet (i): 390, 1979.

CLINICAL PHARMACOLOGY OF INTRAPERITONEAL (IP) BOLUS MITOMYCIN C AND CONTINUOUS IP INFUSION 5-FLUOROURACIL

JOHN W. GYVES, M.D.

INTRODUCTION

Disseminated intraperitoneal (IP) cancer occurs frequently in gastrointestinal and gynecologic malignancies. Malignant ascites can be a major problem in other cancers as well. The pharmacokinetic rationale for IP injection of antineoplastic drugs has been delineated by Dedrick et al.[1] At steady state, the selective advantage (R_d) of a direct drug infusion into the peritoneal cavity relates directly to the total body clearance (TBC) of the drug infused and inversely to the permeability-area product (PA) a measure of peritoneal clearance of the peritoneal surface exposed[1-3]. Initial pilot studies of IP chemotherapy have used 5-fluorouracil (FU),[2, 4] methotrexate,[5, 6] adriamycin,[7] melphalan,[8] and cisplatin[9-11]. These studies have demonstrated that these drugs can be injected IP with acceptable regional toxicity and that the drug concentrations achieved in the peritoneal cavity can be 10- to 1000-fold (1-3 logs) greater than the systemic concentration. Drugs with significant hepatic extraction are ideal, since a portion of such drugs may be metabolized by the liver through portal venous uptake before reaching the systemic circulation. This first-pass effect would be expected to increase the TBC of the drug and maximize the difference between plasma and peritoneal fluid drug concentration.

Previous studies have generally used exchanges of large volumes of drug-containing solutions injected through peritoneal dialysis catheters. Since antimetabolites generally induce cytotoxicity as a function of duration of exposure above critical concentrations,[12] we have investigated the protracted infusion of the antimetabolite FU as a means of selectively sustaining high regional drug levels in the peritoneal cavity and relatively low systemic levels, thus attempting to avoid systemic toxicity. We have also evaluated the regional exposure advantage of IP bolus administration mitomycin C (Mito). Both of these agents have detectable hepatic extraction, although Mito is less avidly extracted by the liver than is FU[13-15]. In addition, to circumvent the inconvenience and morbidity associated with indwelling peritoneal catheters, we have used two totally implanted silastic catheter/port systems that facilitate peritoneal fluid sampling yet obviate the need for maintenance and may avoid the potential infectious complications associated with chronic externalized catheters.

IMPLANTED SYSTEMS AS A MEANS OF IP ACCESS

Based on our favorable experiences with totally implanted venous access devices [16, 17] we have explored the applicability of such systems for peritoneal access. Over the past 2 years, patients eligible for investigational IP chemotherapy protocols at the University of Michigan have undergone the implantation, under local anesthesia, of either an Infus-A-Port (Infusaid, Norwood, MA) (12 pts) or a Port-A-Cath (Pharmacia Nu-Tech, Walpole, MA) (6 pts) attached to a Silastic peritoneal dialysis catheter prior to receiving chemotherapy as previously described[18]. Prior to the availability of such implanted devices, 2 additional patients were treated with the aid of Silastic catheters percutaneously placed at the beginning of each treatment course.

During this 2 year period, 20 patients have received a total of 85 courses (1-9/patient, median 5) of IP FU (1 gm/d x 5 days). In addition, 10 of these patients received a total of 18 courses of Mito. Ten patients had unresectable intra-abdominal cancer and were not eligible for other treatment programs. The remaining patients have been treated as part of an adjuvant protocol for patients with resected Dukes B_2 and C colon cancer. Data obtained from these patients has served to further define the pharmacokinetic advantage of the IP administration of these agents, the relative systemic/regional toxicity involved and the safety of the implanted devices employed.

PRETREATMENT IP VOLUME EXPANSION

The infusion system employed consisted of an IVAC 530 infusion pump (IVAC Corp., San Diego, California), or an IMED 960 infusion pump (IMED Corp., San Diego, California) and Luer-lok extension tubing attached to a Huber-point needle bent at 90° so that the hub of the needle lay parallel to the skin when inserted percutaneously into the port. The needle and adjacent tubing were placed under sterile conditions and secured with Steri-Strips (3M Corp., St. Paul, Minnesota) and Op-Site (Acme United Corp., Bridgeport, Connecticut) for the 5-day infusions. At the completion of an infusion, the needle was removed, and no further maintenance was required. This methodology had been used successfully for continuous intravenous infusions with similar implanted injection port systems[16].

Before therapy with either FU or Mito, 1.5 l lactated Ringers (LR) solution was infused into the abdomen to facilitate drug distribution. This was followed by a constant infusion of LR to maintain this volume. The IP distribution of the fluid was determined by radionuclide scans obtained 1 hour after injection of 1 mCi of Tc99m-sulfur colloid (TcSC) IP[19]. Patients were candidates for pharmacology studies if the scan demonstrated free distribution of the radiopharmaceutical and samples could be readily drawn from the implanted system.

PHARMACOKINETICS OF IP FU INFUSION

The IP infusion therapy consisted of 1 gm FU each day (1 gm FU in 1 l LR infused IP at 42 ml/hr) for 5 days, repeated monthly. Simultaneous peritoneal fluid and venous plasma samples were obtained twice daily beginning 12 hr after initiation of the IP infusion in patients participating in pharmacology studies. Subsequent courses were occasionally given in the outpatient setting (21/85). Under these circumstances, the FU dose was administered in 1 l LR over 1 hour daily x 5.

A total of 85 five-day IP FU infusions were administered in the 20 patients. Seven courses were evaluable for pharmacokinetic studies, and all courses were evaluable for toxicity. FU was assayed by HPLC assay as previously described[18]. The mean plasma FU concentration for individual courses ranged from 0.18 to 1.0 μM. This mean plasma concentration represents the steady-state venous plasma concentration ($C_{SS_{PV}}$). The coefficient of variation for $C_{SS_{PV}}$ in each course ranged from 18% to 68% (mean 30%, median 24%). The mean $C_{SS_{PV}}$ for the entire group was 0.44 μM (median 0.32 μM). The mean peritoneal fluid FU concentration for individual courses ranged from 176 to 2004 μM. The mean concentration over the 5-day infusion represents the steady-state IP FU concentration ($C_{SS_{IP}}$) for that course. The coefficient of variation for $C_{SS_{IP}}$ for individual courses ranged from 9% to 43% (mean 27%, median 27%). The mean $C_{SS_{IP}}$ for the entire group was 622 μM (median 475 μM).

Total body clearance (TBC) was calculated from the ratio of the constant infusion dose rate and the venous plasma steady-state concentration. In these seven treatment courses, TBC averaged 16.5 l/min (median 16.6 l/min). The permeability area product (PA) was determined from steady-state levels ($C_{SS_{PV}}$ and $C_{SS_{IP}}$) and the TBC[2]. The mean PA in these patients was 16.1 ml/min (median 11.1 ml/min). The selective regional advantage (R_d) of IP infusion FU was directly determined as the ratio of $C_{SS_{IP}}$ to $C_{SS_{PV}}$ and also calculated from values derived for TBC and PA[1, 3]. Both methods gave equivalent results. In these patients the mean R_d was 2218 (median 1023).

In addition to the 5-day IP infusion, one patient received a 24-hr IV infusion of FU (1 gm/24 hr) after the abdomen was loaded as described for the IP infusion treatment. LR was infused IP to maintain this volume during the IV infusion. Peritoneal fluid and venous blood samples were obtained during the infusion and assayed for FU. Based on the formula derived by Collins et al.,[20] the extraction of FU by the liver and peritoneal surface was calculated from steady-state venous plasma levels obtained from the intravenous and subsequent IP infusion. In this case the extraction of FU was found to be 75%. The TBC during the 24-hr intravenous infusion was 5.9 l/min, which is similar to that previously reported[21].

TBC for this patient during two separate IP infusion courses was 16.6 and 24.1 l/min. This difference in TBC is consistent with the regional extraction noted.

On a separate treatment course, one patient received a single IP bolus of FU (1 gm) for comparison with the IP infusion kinetic data. The abdomen was loaded with fluid and the LR infused as described above before injection of the FU. Peritoneal fluid and venous plasma samples were obtained over 16 hr and were assayed for FU. The TBC of 14.3 l/min for this patient given the IP Bolus is similar to that reported[2]. The TBC was 29.5 l/min during the 5-day IP infusion in the same patient. Thus, the improved regional advantage of IP FU infusion results, in part, from a maximized TBC compared to that seen with IP bolus or IV infusion FU.

TOXICITY OF IP INFUSION OF FU

The 6 patients received a total of 25 IP infusions of FU. Toxicity was minimal. There was no evidence of systemic toxicity (mucositis or myelosuppression), but all patients experienced mild abdominal discomfort related to the fluid volume infused, i.e., from fluid loading before the FU infusion. Symptomatic chemical peritonitis (6 episodes) occurred in 3 patients who received a total of 12 courses. Peritoneal fluid was sampled on the third day of each infusion for cell count, differential, and bacterial culture, and evidence of mild sterile inflammatory reaction was present in most patients. There were no infectious complications.

PHARMACOKINETICS OF IP BOLUS MITOMYCIN C

A total of 18 courses of IP Mito were administered in 10 patients. The early Phase I experience suggested that 10 mg given as a 1-minute bolus injection was the maximum dose tolerated. Seven courses in 3 patients who received this dose were evaluable for pharmacokinetic studies, and all courses were evaluable for toxicity. The mean IP exposure advantage ($AUC_{IP_{0\to\infty}}/AUC_{PV_{0\to\infty}}$) for bolus Mito administration was 31.8 (range 16.1 - 84.5). The regional advantage, as measured by the ratio of peak IP and plasma drug concentrations achieved, averaged 82.3. The mean TBC was .672 l/min (range .375-.940), and the elimination half-life averaged almost 3 hours (range 1.2-5.4)[22].

TOXICITY OF IP BOLUS MITO

Three patients received 7 IP bolus injections of Mito (10 mg). There was no evidence of systemic toxicity (mucositis or myelosuppression), but all patients experienced mild abdominal discomfort with the treatment. Symptomatic chemical peritonitis occurred in 5 of the 7 courses, and analysis of peritoneal fluid demonstrated mild sterile inflammatory reactions in these cases. There was no change in the distribution of IP fluid as determined by TcSC scans in those who received more than one course.

CONCLUSION

Continuous intraperitoneal infusion of FU results in a 2-3 log regional to systemic exposure advantage, which can be maintained over 5 days. Twenty patients received a total of 67 courses of IP FU alone. Eighteen courses (27%) were accompanied by symptomatic chemical peritonitis. Ten patients have received a total of 18 courses of IP Mito (5-30 mg) followed by the 5-day FU infusion. Symptomatic chemical peritonitis has been dose limiting (MTD Mito 10 mg) with 60% of patients experiencing this toxicity at this dose. The data presented suggests a 2-log difference in peak drug concentration and regional exposure (AUC) for the IP route at this dose. Finally, the totally implanted catheter-port systems employed in these treatments appear to facilitate IP drug administration without the risk of catheter-related infections commonly seen with external catheters.

REFERENCES

1. Dedrick RL, Myers CE, Bungay PM, DeVita VT: Pharmacokinetic rationale for peritoneal drug administration in the treatment of ovarian cancer. Cancer treat Rep (62):1-11, 1978.
2. Speyer JL, Collins JM, Dedrick RL, Brennan MF, Buckpitt AR, Londer H, DeVita Vt, Myers CE: Phase I and pharmacological studies of 5-fluorouracil administered intraperitoneally. Cancer Res (40):567-572, 1980.
3. Ensminger WD, Gyves JW: Regional cancer chemotherapy. Cancer Treat Rep (68):101-115, 1984.
4. Speyer JL, Sugarbaker PH, Collins JM, Dedrick RL, Klecker RW Jr, Myers CE: Portal levels and hepatic clearance of 5-fluorouracil after intraperitoneal administration in humans. Cancer Res (41):1916-1922, 1981.
5. Howell SB, Chu BBF, Wung WE, Metha BM, Mendelsohn J: Long-duration intracavitary infusion of methotrexate with systemic leucovorin protection in patients with malignant effusions. J Clin Invest (67):1161-1170, 1981.
6. Jones RB, Collins JM, Myers CE, Brooks AE, Hubbard SM, Balow JE, Brennan MF, Dedrick RL, DeVita VT: High-volume intraperitoneal chemotherapy with methotrexate in patients with cancer. Cancer Res (41):55-59, 1981.

INTRAPERITONEAL ADRIAMYCIN AND 5-FLUOROURACIL IN OVARIAN CANCER

R.F. OZOLS, R.C. YOUNG AND C.E. MYERS

Medicine (RFO, RCY) and Clinical Pharmacology (CEM) Branches, Division of Cancer Treatment, National Cancer Institute, Bethesda, MD

I. INTRODUCTION

Drug resistance, both intrinsic resistance present in many previously untreated patients and acquired resistance, which frequently develops in patients who respond to therapy, is a major clinical problem in ovarian cancer which limits the overall effectiveness of most chemotherapeutic agents. An understanding of the mechanisms responsible for resistance in ovarian cancer would likely facilitate pharmacologic attempts to reverse or modify this resistance and thereby increase the efficacy of these drugs. Intraperitoneal chemotherapy in ovarian cancer is an attempt to overcome drug resistance which results from the inability to achieve cytotoxic drug levels in the peritoneal cavity following either oral or intravenous administration of the same drugs. The pharmacologic rationale for intraperitoneal administration of anticancer agents has been presented elsewhere in this monograph by Collins et al. The characteristics of an appropriate drug for intraperitoneal administration in ovarian cancer are summarized in Table 1.

Table 1

Characteristics of a Suitable Drug For Intraperitoneal Chemotherapy

1. Slow clearance from peritoneal cavity compared to clearance from blood, which leads to a marked pharmacologic advantage (high ratio of peak peritoneal drug levels to peak blood levels).
2. The drug must produce a tolerable degree of peritoneal irritation.
3. Cytotoxic peritoneal concentrations of drug should be achieved.
4. The drug should diffuse into intraabdominal tumor masses.

Pharmacologic modelling studies predict that the optimal pharmacologic advantage will be achieved with repetitive dialysis and with the drug delivered in a large volume of dialysate to ensure uniform distribution throughout the peritoneal cavity (1). In order to facilitate such a schedule of intraperitoneal drug delivery,the Clinical Pharmacology and Medicine Branches, NCI, have extensively used semi-permanent indwelling Tenckhoff dialysis catheters in patients with ovarian cancer. These catheters provide continuous access to the peritoneal cavity and permit large volume (2 L) exchanges of drug-containing dialysate. Phase I trials of intraperitoneal methotrexate (2), 5-Fluorouracil (3) and Adriamycin (4) have been completed in ovarian cancer patients, as has a phase II trial of intraperitoneal 5-Fluorouracil (5). A phase II trial of intraperitoneal Adriamycin is still in progress.

II. TENCKHOFF CATHETERS

The technical considerations in the use of Tenckhoff catheters for intraperitoneal chemotherapy in 78 patients at the NCI have recently been reviewed (6). In 66/78 patients the catheters were implanted under local anesthesia through the anterior abdominal wall. The catheters have a Dacron, polyester fiber, cuff that is embedded in the subcutaneous tissue,and the subsequent fibrous reaction forms a barrier to infectious organisms. Complications of catheter placement were infrequent; however, intestinal perforation did occur in 3/78 (4%) of patients. Minor complications included: transient minor intraperitoneal bleeding, pain at the incision site lasting 4-6 days, and transient leakage at the catheter site until the exit site healed.

The most significant threat to catheter maintenance was infection. There were 3 cases of documented intraabdominal sepsis in the 78 patients. The overall incidence of catheter-related peritonitis was 10 percent per catheter year.

The majority of catheters functioned without obstruction to inflow or drainage. When difficulty to inflow was encountered, it was frequently the result of a fibrous plug, which was usually cleared using forceful irrigation. Occasionally, if simple irrigation did not relieve the obstruction, repositioning of the catheter was required. When these techniques were used to maintain catheter patency, there were only 5 patients in whom retention of dialysis required major alterations in the schedule of drug delivery.

III. PHASE I TRIALS OF INTRAPERITONEAL CHEMOTHERAPY

Table 2 summarizes the results of phase I trials of intraperitoneal methotrexate, 5-Fluorouracil, and Adriamycin in relapsed ovarian cancer patients. Methotrexate was the initial drug evaluated at the NCI (2).A pharmacologic advantage was achieved with intermittent intraperitoneal dialysis. However, the local toxicity of peritoneal irritation was severe, and since objective responses were not observed, methotrexate was replaced by more active agents.

Table 2

Phase I Trials of Intraperitoneal Chemotherapy in Ovarian Cancer

Drug	No. Patients	Schedule	Pharmacologic[a] Advantage	Dose-limiting Toxicity[b]
Methotrexate (Ref 2)	5	50 uM:8x4 hr exchanges q 2 wks	18-36	Peritonitis
5-Fluorouracil (Ref 3)	10	4 mM:8x4 hr exchanges q 2 wk	298	Myelosuppression Mucositis
Adriamycin (Ref 4)	10	36 uM:4 hr dwell q 2 wks	474	Abdominal Pain

[a] Ratio of peak intraperitoneal level to peak plasma level.
[b] Common toxicities, although not dose-limiting, were: methotrexate (myelosuppression); 5-Fluorouracil (abdominal pain); Adriamycin (mild nausea and vomiting and mild myelosuppression).

In the phase I trial of intraperitoneal 5-Fluorouracil, myelosuppression and mucositis were the dose-limiting toxicities (3). A marked pharmacologic advantage of 298 was achieved with repetitive 4-hour exchanges of 4 mM 5-Fluorouracil.

The results of the phase I trial of intraperitoneal Adriamycin have recently been reported (4). Adriamycin has several features which make it a potentially useful drug for intraperitoneal chemotherapy in ovarian cancer. (1) It is an active drug with a response rate of 40% in previously untreated patients; (2) its pharmacologic properties (high molecular weight and hydrophilicity) predict for slow peritoneal clearance; (3) the intraperitoneal route of administration was demonstrated to be markedly superior to intravenous Adriamycin in a murine model of ovarian cancer (7,8); (4) dose-response relationships between Adriamycin and *in vitro* cytotoxcity to human ovarian cancer cells obtained from patient biopsies or malignant ascites have identified a subset of patients in whom intraperitoneal Adriamycin would be of potential benefit (9,10). Ovarian cancer cells obtained from patients who were refractory to a non-Adriamycin-containing drug regimen were resistant in the colony-forming assay to concentrations of Adriamycin achievable by intravenous administration. However, when these same cells were exposed to a concentration of Adriamycin which was 10 times higher than the peak level after intravenous administration, and which was potentially achievable by intraperitoneal administration of Adriamycin, marked cytotoxicity (less than 20% colony survival) was observed. In contrast, cells obtained from patients who were clinically resistant to intravenous Adriamycin were also resistant *in vitro* after exposure to Adriamycin concentrations potentially achievable by intraperitoneal administration. These *in vitro* studies were consistent with the low response rate of intravenous Adriamycin in previously treated patients (11) and suggested that intraperitoneal chemotherapy with Adriamycin may be of benefit to patients who have not become clinically resistant to intravenous Adriamycin.

In the phase I trial,10 patients who were refractory to non-Adriamycin-containing combination chemotherapy regimens were treated with intraperitoneal Adriamycin at concentrations ranging from 9 to 54 uM. Adriamycin was administered every two weeks in 2L of heparin-free dialysate (to prevent precipitation of Adriamycin) with a 4-hour dwell time. The dose-limiting toxicity in this phase I trial was a dose-dependent sterile peritonitis, table 3.

Table 3

Peritoneal Toxicity of Intraperitoneal Adriamycin[a]

Adriamycin Concentration in Dialysate	Peritoneal Irritation: Pain Intensity[b] (per cycle) +	++	+++	Sterile Ascites	Formation of Adhesions
9 uM	1/3				
18 uM	2/5				
36 uM	9/17	5/17	2/17		
45 uM		4/17	3/7	1/7	
54 uM		2/6	4/6	1/6	2/6

[a] From Ref 4.
[b] Pain intensity: + = persisting for less than 24 hours; ++ = 1-3 days of pain requiring mild analgesics; +++ = pain persisting for 3-8 days requiring codeine analgesia.

In the phase I trial of intraperitoneal Adriamycin, there were 3 objective responses. One patient had a negative second-look peritoneoscopy after 6 cycles of therapy [peak dose 54 uM]. A subsequent peritoneoscopy 18 months later revealed malignant cells in the peritoneal washings. A second patient with multiple small peritoneal implants received 6 cycles of intraperitoneal Adriamycin [peak dose 45 uM] after which only a single focus of malignant cells was found in the omentum. A third patient whose only evidence for residual disease was malignant cells in peritoneal washings developed negative cytologic washings, which persisted for 4 months after intraperitoneal Adriamycin. Two additional patients with bulky disease had a marked decrease in ascites production while on therapy with intraperitoneal Adriamycin.

The clinical activity of Adriamycin in this trial was likely the result of anti-tumor activity and not merely a sclerotic effect. The decrease in ascites was accompanied by a decrease in the actual number of malignant cells obtained from the abdominal cavity. In addition, malignant cells obtained from the peritoneal cavity immediately after therapy with intraperitoneal Adriamycin no longer were able to proliferate, as documented by the absence of colony formation in the stem cell assay (4).

Adriamycin concentrations were measured using an HPLC assay. The maximum pharmacologic advantage was 474, and this was higher than observed with either methotrexate (18-36) or 5-Fluorouracil (298). The peak plasma levels of Adriamycin after a 60 mg/2L intraperitoneal dose were 10 times lower than after a 60 mg intravenous dose of Adriamycin. The levels of Adriamycin required for in vitro cytotoxicity against cells obtained from patients who were refractory to non-Adriamycin-containing regimens were achieved intraperitoneally in these patients.

IV. PHASE II TRIAL OF INTRAPERITONEAL 5-FLUOROURACIL

The results of a phase II trial of intraperitoneal 5-Fluorouracil in ovarian cancer patients have recently been reported (5). Table 4 summarizes the patient characteristics and the schedule of administration. A total of 69 cycles of intraperitoneal 5-Fluorouracil was administered to 14 previously treated patients (12 of whom had received prior intravenous 5-Fluorouracil). The median number of cycles of intraperitoneal 5-Fluorouracil per patient was 6.

One patient in this trial had an objective response to intraperitoneal 5-Fluorouracil. This patient had multiple 1-2 cm nodules throughout the peritoneum prior to therapy, and after 5 cycles of intraperitoneal 5-Fluorouracil no tumor was found at a second-look laparotomy. This was the only patient treated with intraperitoneal 5-Fluorouracil in which an objective response was observed, resulting in a response rate of 7%.

Table 4

Phase II Trial of Intraperitoneal 5-Fluorouracil (Ref 5)

Patient Characteristics	
No. Patients	14
Previously Treated	14
Prior i.v. 5-FU	12
Bulky (> 2 cm masses)	6
Non Bulky (< 2 cm masses)	8
Drug Therapy	
Concentration:	4mM 5-FU dissolved in 2L of Inpersol containing 1.5% dextrose to which was added 1000 units heparin, 8 meq KCL, and 50 meq $NaHCO_3$.
Schedule:	Dwell time of 4 hours and a total of 8 exchanges (drainage and filling time 30 minutes) performed with each 36-hour course of treatment. Repeat every 14 days until disease progression or severe toxicity.

Six patients had bulky disease prior to therapy, and 4 of these patients developed intraabdominal progression of disease while on therapy with intraperitoneal 5-Fluorouracil. The other 2 patients developed disease progression in extraperitoneal sites.

Of the 8 patients who had small volume disease at the time intraperitoneal 5-Fluorouracil was started, only one patient developed progression of intraabdominal disease while on therapy. Those patients who had disease stablization after 6 cycles of intraperitoneal 5-Fluorouracil received alternate therapies due to the development of persistent abdominal pain.

The toxicity of intraperitoneal 5-Fluorouracil in this trial is summarized in Table 5. While myelosuppression, nausea and vomiting, and mucositis were common, the degree of these toxicities was not severe. Abdominal pain, however,was the major toxicity of intraperitoneal 5-Flurorouracil. Fifty percent of the patients had severe abdominal pain with at least one cycle of therapy. The presence of abdominal pain even in patients who had small volume of disease at the time therapy was started strongly indicates that the therapy, and not the disease itself, was responsible for the abdominal discomfort associated with intraperitoneal 5-Fluorouracil.

Table 5
Toxicity of Intraperitoneal 5-Fluorouracil in Refractory Ovarian Cancer Patients (Ref 5)

Toxicity	Incidence
Hematologic Suppression	
WBC < 1000 ul	14%
Platelets < 1000 ul	27%
Hemoglobin > 2 g/dl decrease	7%
Nausea and Vomiting	
Mild	29%
Moderate	67%
Mucositis	
Mild	29%
Moderate	7%
Abdominal Pain	
Mild	7%
Moderate	36%
Severe	50%

V. PHASE II TRIAL OF INTRAPERITONEAL ADRIAMYCIN

A phase II trail of intraperitoneal Adriamycin is in progress at the NCI. The details of the trial are summarized in Table 6. On the basis of responses in the phase I trial in patients with small volume disease only, patients with bulky disease are not eligible for this study. In addition, patients must not have received prior Adriamycin therapy since the dose-response relationships to Adriamycin in cells from these patients do not suggest that the increased Adriamycin levels in the peritoneum after intraperitoneal therapy will be sufficient to produce a significant increase in cytotoxicity (10).

Five patients currently are evaluable for response. Two patients had no clinical evidence of disease after 6 cycles of intraperitoneal Adriamycin, but second-look laparotomies were not done. One of the patients subsequently relapsed in the brain. It is interesting to note, however, that she did not have clinical evidence of intraperitoneal disease at the time of CNS relapse.

Abdominal pain is the major toxicity of intraperitoneal Adriamycin. The majority of cycles have had to be increased from two weeks to three weeks to allow for the pain to completely disappear. Systemic steroids administered for 24 hours before and after intraperitoneal Adriamycin have not markedly reduced the abdominal pain.

Table 6

Phase II Trial of Intraperitoneal Adriamycin in Ovarian Cancer

I. Patient Eligibility
   A. Residual small volume (< 2 cm masses) after induction chemotherapy.
   B. No prior therapy with intravenous Adriamycin.

II. Schedule
   A. Adriamycin Dose: 40 mg/2L dialysate with a 4-hour dwell administered every 2 weeks for 6 cycles of treatment.
   B. Dose Modification: Increase length of time between cycles for severe abdominal pain and decrease dose if abdominal pain still persists.

III. Preliminary Results
   A. Five patients have been treated: 2 patients without clinical evidence of disease after therapy,but second-look laparotomy not performed. One patient relapsed with brain metastases after 18 months.
   B. Toxicity: Abdominal pain severe. Interval between treatments increased to 3 weeks in 40% of cycles. Steroids have not eliminated pain.

Since the dose-limiting toxicity of intraperitoneal Adriamycin is a sterile peritonitis, an anthracycline analog which has the same spectrum of activity against ovarian cancer as does Adriamycin, but which does not produce the same degree of peritoneal irritation,may be a more suitable drug for intraperitoneal use. We have demonstrated that aclacinomycin, an Adriamycin analog which does not produce tissue necrosis when extravasated into soft tissue, has a similar dose-response relationship to cytotoxicity in human ovarian cancer cell lines as does Adriamycin (12). Since it may not have the same degree of peritoneal toxicity as Adriamycin, it may be a more useful anthracycline for intraperitoneal therapy.

DISCUSSION

The phase I-II trials of intraperitoneal chemotherapy have demonstrated the feasibility and safety of intermittent, large-volume dialysis with semi-permanent Tenckhoff catheters in ovarian cancer patients, including those patients who have had multiple previous surgical procedures and who have a large volume of bulky disease. In addition, the intraperitoneal administration of chemotherapeutic agents has produced a marked pharmacologic advantage. The peak levels in the peritoneal cavity have been 18-474 times greater than the peak plasma levels, table 3. However, the therapeutic benefit of intraperitoneal chemotherapy and the optimum clinical situations for its use have not been established.

From the phase I trial in which objective responses were seen in patients with small volume disease only, and from experimental studies demonstrating that Adriamycin penetrated into the outermost 4-6 cell layers of intraabdominal tumor masses in a murine model of ovarian cancer (7), it does not appear likely that intraperitoneal Adriamycin will be of benefit in patients with bulky disease. The absence of any objective responses to intraperitoneal 5-Fluorouracil in the phase II trial in patients who had received prior intravenous therapy with 5-Fluorouracil indicates that intraperitoneal 5-Fluorouracil be further evaluated only in those patients who are not resistant to intravenous 5-Fluorouracil. Similarly, the nature of the dose-response relationship to Adriamycin in cells obtained from ovarian cancer patients who were refractory to Adriamycin-containing drug regimens likewise suggests that intraperitoneal Adriamycin will not be clinically beneficial in patients who are resistant to intravenous Adriamycin (10).

Table 7 summarizes those clinical situations where intraperitoneal 5-Fluorouracil or intraperitoneal Adriamycin may be of benefit in the treatment of patients with ovarian cancer. Studies currently are in progress at the Medicine Branch, NCI and by the Gynecology-Oncology Group of intraperitoneal chemotherapy in patients who have small volume residual disease after induction chemotherapy. In addition, the role of maintenance therapy aimed at preventing late relapses in patients who achieve a pathologically confirmed complete remission is

Table 7

Potential Role of Intraperitoneal Adriamycin or 5-Fluorouracil in the Treatment of Ovarian Cancer

I. Early Stage Disease
   A. As an adjuvant to surgery in high-risk patients.
II. Advanced Stage Disease
   A. Small volume residual disease after surgery.
   B. Small volume residual disease after systemic induction chemotherapy.
   C. As maintenance (consolidation) therapy in patients who achieve a complete remission.
   D. Combined with systemic chemotherapy as part of an intensive induction regimen.

also under investigation at the Medicine Branch (13). The overall benefit of intraperitoneal chemotherapy in the treatment of ovarian cancer will be established by these and other clinical trials.

In addition to intraperitoneal chemotherapy, alternative pharmacologic techniques are under study which have the potential to increase the efficacy of certain chemotherapeutic agents, and in some cases, reverse acquired drug resistance. Nephrotoxicity is no longer the dose-limiting toxicity of cisplatin when cisplatin is adminstered in hypertonic saline with a vigorous chloruresis (14). Intravenous high-dose cisplatin has been shown to have a 40% response rate in ovarian cancer patients who have had progressive disease after standard dose cisplatin. High-dose cisplatin is currently under evaluation in previously untreated ovarian cancer patients at the Medicine Branch, NCI. Verapamil, a calcium channel blocker,has been shown to reverse Adriamycin resistance in some human ovarian cancer cell lines (15), and a trial of verapamil plus Adriamycin in refractory ovarian cancer patients is also in progress at the Medicine Branch, NCI (16).

Finally, alkylating agent cytotoxicity has been shown to be a function of glutathione levels in ovarian cancer cell lines (17). Pharmacologic depletion of glutathione levels with an inhibitor of glutathione synthesis leads to reversal of melphalan resistance _in vitro_. These studies indicate that certain agents which increase the cytotoxicity of anticancer drugs may be useful in both the systemic and intraperitoneal chemotherapy of ovarian cancer.

REFERENCES

1. Dedrick RL, Myers CE, Bugnay PM, DeVita VT: Pharmacokinetic rationale for peritoneal drug administration in treatment of ovarian cancer. Cancer Treat Rep (62):1-11, 1978.

2. Jones RB, Collins JM, Myers CE, Brooks AE, Hubbard SM, Ballow JW, Brennan MF, Dedrick RL, DeVita VT: High-volume intraperitoneal chemotherapy with methotrexate in patients with cancer. Cancer Res (41):55-59, 1981.

3. Speyer JL, Collins JM, Dedrick RL, Brennan MF, Londer H, DeVita VT, Myers CM: Phase I and pharmacologic studies of 5-Fluorouracil administered intraperitoneally. Cancer Res (40):567-572, 1980.

4. Ozols RF, Young RC, Speyer JL, Sugarbaker PH, Greene R, Jenkins J, Myers CE: Phase I and pharmacologic studies of Adriamycin administered intraperitoneally to patients with ovarian cancer. Cancer Res (42):4265-4269, 1982.

5. Ozols RF, Speyer JL, Jenkins J,Myers CE: Phase II trial of 5-Fluorouracil administered intraperitoneally to patients with refractory ovarian cancer. Cancer Treat Rep (in press) 1984.

6. Jenkins J, Sugarbaker PH, Gianola FJ, Myers CE: Technical considerations in the use of intraperitoneal chemotherapy administered by Tenckhoff catheter. Surgery (154):858-864, 1982.

7. Ozols RF, Grotzinger KR, Fisher RI, Myers CE, Young RC: Kinetic characterization and response to chemotherapy in a transplantable murine ovarian cancer. Cancer Res (39):3202-3208, 1979.

8. Ozols RF, Locker GY, Doroshow JH, Grotzinger KR, Myers CE, Young RC: Pharmacokinetics of Adriamycin and tissue penetration in murine ovarian cancer. Cancer Res (30):3209-3214, 1979.

9. Ozols RF, Willson JKV, Grotzinger KR, Young RC: Cloning of human ovarian cancer cells in soft agar from malignant effusions and peritoneal washings. Cancer Res (40):2743-2747, 1980.

10. Ozols RF, Willson JKV, Weltz MD, Grotzinger KR, Myers CE, Young RC: Inhibition of human ovarian cancer colony formation by Adriamycin and its major metabolites. Cancer Res (40):4109-4112, 1980.

11. Hubbard SM, Barkes P, Young RC: Adriamycin therapy for advanced ovarian carcinoma recurrent after chemotherapy. Cancer Treat Rep (67):1375-1377, 1978.

12. Ozols RF, Myers CE, Young RC: The potential role of anthracyclines in the intraperitoneal chemotherapy of ovarian cancer. In: Hansen HH (ed). Anthracyclines and Cancer Therapy. Excerpta Medica Amsterdam, 1983, 158-165.

13. Young RC, Howser DM, Myers CE, Ozols RF, Fisher RI, Wesley M, Chabner BA: Combination chemotherapy (CHEX-UP) with intraperitoneal maintenance in advanced ovarian adenocarcinoma. Proc Amer Soc Clin Oncol (22):465, 1981.

14. Ozols RF, Corden BJ, Jacob J, Wesley MN, Ostchega Y,Young RC: High-dose cisplatin in hypertonic saline. Annals Int Med (100):19-24, 1984.

15. Rogan AM, Hamilton TC, Young RC, Ozols RF: Pharmacologic modulation of Adriamycin resistance in ovarian cancer. In: Salmon S (ed). Proc IV Tumor Cloning Conf (in press) 1984.

16. Ozols RF, Rogan AM, Hamilton TC, Klecker R, Young RC: Verapamil plus Adriamycin in refractory ovarian cancer: design of a clinical trial on basis of reversal of Adriamycin resistance in human ovarian cancer cell lines. Proc Amer Assoc Cancer Res (in press) 1984.

17. Ozols RF, Green JA, Hamilton TC, Vistica DT, Young RC: Potentiation of melphalan cytotoxicity in human ovarian cancer cell lines. In: Salmon S (ed). Proc IV Tumor Cloning Conf (in press) 1984.

COMBINATION CISPLATIN-BASED INTRACAVITARY CHEMOTHERAPY

MAURIE MARKMAN, M.D.

The simultaneous administration of several chemotherapeutic agents individually active against a particular neoplasm has become a major therapeutic principle in clinical oncology. The advantages of such an approach include the ability to administer drugs which are potentially non-cross resistant and which demonstrate non-overlapping toxicities. It has been hypothesized that the administration of combination chemotherapy will help prevent the emergence of a multiply resistant cell line to which all antineoplastic agents are inactive (1). The success of combination chemotherapy in increasing the complete remission rate, prolonging survival and curing a significant percentage of patients with childhood acute lymphoblastic leukemia, Hodgkin's disease, diffuse histiocytic lymphoma and testicular carcinoma attests to the soundness of the basic principles of multi-agent chemotherapy. In addition, in certain other malignancies where the cure rate remains poor, significant palliation of symptoms and prolongation of survival can be achieved through the use of combination chemotherapy.

For certain tumors, however, there has been legitimate concern that the injection of chemotherapeutic agents intravenously may not be the optimal way to get drug to tumor. While this is certainly the case for tumors "protected" by the blood-brain barrier, it also might be true for neoplasms largely confined to extravascular cavities. While most drugs have access to the well-vascularized marrow and gut following intravenous injection, they have less ability to enter tumor located in body cavities because of longer diffusional distances. Pharmacological modeling has suggested a significant advantage for the intracavitary administration of certain chemotherapeutic agents compared to the same drug administered systemically (2). Phase I trials have demonstrated the pharmacokinetic advantage, safety, and clinical efficacy of several drugs administered as single agents via the intraperitoneal route, including cisplatin (3), cytarabine (4), doxorubicin (5), 5-fluorouracil (6), melphalan (7), methotrexate (8,9) and mitomycin (10).

The intracavitary chemotherapy program at the UCSD Cancer Center has focused much of its attention on the development of an effective combination intraperitoneal chemotherapy program for ovarian carcinoma. In spite of the significant sensitivity of this neoplasm to several agents and reported complete clinical response rates for patients with advanced disease approaching 60% utilizing cisplatin-based combination chemotherapeutic regimens, the vast majority of women with ovarian carcinoma will eventually die of their disease (11-13). However, even in its advanced stages this tumor tends to remain localized to the abdominal cavity. This factor and the demonstration that several active agents in ovarian carcinoma have shown a major pharmacokinetic advantage for the abdominal cavity when administered via the intraperitoneal route make this an ideal tumor to which to attempt to administer high-dose intracavitary chemotherapy.

Our initial combination intraperitoneal chemotherapy program investigated the administration of cisplatin, doxorubicin, and cytarabine. Previous work at our institution had demonstrated that cisplatin could be administered intraperitoneally at doses up to 270 mg/m^2 when sodium thiosulfate was simultaneously infused intravenously to protect against cisplatin-induced nephrotoxicity (3). The peak peritoneal drug concentration of free reactive cisplatin averaged 21-fold higher than in the plasma, and the area under the peritoneal cavity cisplatin elimination curve averaged 12-fold higher than under the plasma curve. Perhaps most importantly, however, at maximally tolerated doses of cisplatin (270 mg/m^2) administered along with sodium thiosulfate, the systemic exposure to cisplatin was twofold higher than with intravenous drug administration (100 mg/m^2) (3). Thus, the intraperitoneal administration of this agent not only allowed for significantly higher local concentrations (direct tumor-drug interactions) but also exposed tumor to as much cisplatin via capillary flow as when the drug was administered intravenously.

Doxorubicin was added to the intraperitoneal chemotherapy regimen as it has been shown to be one of the most active agents against ovarian carcinoma. In addition, cisplatin/doxorubicin combination chemotherapy has demonstrated among the highest overall and complete response rates reported in this disease (13). Finally, investigators at the National Cancer Institute have previously demonstrated objective responses to this agent administered intraperitoneally to patients with ovarian carcinoma failing front-line chemotherapy (5).

Cytarabine was selected as the third agent in our initial combination regimen. Until recently this drug had been believed to have minimal activity against solid tumors in general and ovarian carcinoma in particular (14). However, the safety, pharmacokinetic advantage, and efficacy of this agent in ovarian carcinoma when administered intraperitoneally has now been demonstrated (4). In addition, several tumors tested from individuals with ovarian carcinoma in an *in vitro* clonogenic assay were found to be sensitive to cytarabine only at concentrations greater than that which could be achieved safely by systemic drug administration, but which could be achieved safely by intraperitoneal administration of the agent. Finally, recent observations of dramatic synergy demonstrated *in vitro* between cisplatin and cytarabine against LoVo cells (a human colon carcinoma cell line) has sparked considerable interest in the potential clinical application of this laboratory phenomenon (15,16). In particular, this synergy was shown to be highly concentration-dependent, with a remarkable 1,600-fold increased cell kill noted at a cytarabine concentration of 4×10^{-2}M. While this concentration could clearly not be safely achieved in humans through the intravenous administration of cytarabine, it could conceivably be reached for some finite period of time during the intraperitoneal administration of the agent.

Following initial *in vitro* stability studies of the three-drug mixture in solution, a phase I trial of escalating dosages of the drug combination was instituted in patients with refractory ovarian carcinoma or in individuals with other malignancies principally localized to the abdominal cavity. Prior to the institution of therapy, all patients without medical contraindications had a semi-permanent indwelling catheter placed into the peritoneal cavity through which the drugs were administered. In selected patients unable or unwilling to have a catheter placed surgically, treatment was administered by percutaneous placement of a peritoneal dialysis catheter with each treatment course. Treatment was generally initiated 7-14 days following catheter placement to allow for adequate wound healing.

The drugs to be administered were mixed together and instilled intraperitoneally in two liters of normal saline. Following a four-hour dwell time, as much of the remaining fluid as possible was removed. In addition to overnight hydration, patients received sodium thiosulfate both as an intravenous bolus (4 grams/m^2 in 250 ml of sterile water) and an infusion (12 grams/m^2 in 1 liter sterile water over six hours), starting at the time of intraperitoneal drug administration. Treatment was repeated at 28 day intervals.

During this phase I trial, the dose of cisplatin was increased from 100 mg/m^2 to 200 mg/m^2 while the dose of cytarabine was escalated from 50 mg (10^{-4}M) to 490 mg (10^{-3}M). Based upon a previously reported phase I trial of single agent doxorubicin administered intraperitoneally, a dose of 20 mg/2L treatment volume (18 μM) was selected (5). Unfortunately, this dose of doxorubicin was found to cause excessive local abdominal discomfort, with 60% of treatment courses at this dose level being associated with pain lasting longer than 72 hours or requiring narcotic analgesia. With a dose reduction of doxorubicin to 2 mg/2L (2 μM), the incidence of moderate to severe pain decreased to 10%-20% of treatment courses.

Nephrotoxicity was not excessive with serum creatinine rises to >2.0 mg/dl occurring during only 8% of courses administered at the 200 mg/m^2 dose of cisplatin. There was no evidence of nephrotoxicity at the 100 mg/m^2 cisplatin dose level. The only patients exhibiting any evidence of nephrotoxicity had previously been heavily pre-treated with intravenous cisplatin. In addition, in all cases the serum creatinine returned to baseline within six weeks of therapy.

Myelosuppression was also mild during this clinical trial. Only four of 101 courses were associated with white blood cell count depressions of <2,000/mm^3, while following three courses the platelet count dropped to <75,000/mm^3. Of note is the fact that all but one case of significant bone marrow depression occurred with the administration of 20 mg of doxorubicin along with cisplatin administered at the 200 mg/m^2

dose level. No patient required hospitalization for complications related to leukopenia or thrombocytopenia.

Nausea and vomiting were not well controlled in spite of intensive combination antiemetic therapy. However, no patient withdrew from treatment because of this problem. One patient experienced an exacerbation of a cisplatin-induced peripheral neuropathy. There were no other episodes of neuropathy observed during this trial. A single episode of bacterial peritonitis developed in association with placement of a percutaneous dialysis catheter. There were no other infectious complications documented during this study, nor were there any problems related to Tenckhoff catheter placement.

Of the 31 patients treated in this trial, 20 are evaluable for response to therapy. Eleven patients, although having documented residual or recurrent tumor, had no measurable disease. Eight patients exhibited objective responses, including seven of 15 patients (47%) with ovarian carcinoma. Responses included disappearance or marked decrease in ascites in four patients, decrease in a vaginal wall mass in one patient, and conversion of positive peritoneal cytology to negative in two patients. One patient achieved a clinical complete remission lasting seven months. Additionally, one patient requiring an exploratory laparotomy for bowel obstruction was found to be pathologically free of tumor. Extensive adhesions believed to be secondary to doxorubicin were found at surgery and were felt to be the cause of the obstruction.

In summary, in this trial we demonstrated the efficacy of combination intraperitoneal chemotherapy with cisplatin, cytarabine and doxorubicin in refractory ovarian carcinoma. In addition, one patient with diffuse carcinomatosis from an adenocarcinoma of unknown primary presenting with partial small bowel obstruction achieved a dramatic partial remission with relief of his pain and obstruction lasting 10 months. Unfortunately, in this trial using combination therapy, local abdominal discomfort from the doxorubicin was unacceptable, particularly at the 20 mg/2L (18 μM) dose level.

In an effort to take additional advantage of the potential _in vivo_ synergy between cisplatin and cytarabine and to avoid the problem of doxorubicin-induced chemical peritonitis, we instituted a trial of combination intraperitoneal chemotherapy with cisplatin (100-200 mg/m^2)

and a significantly increased concentration of cytarabine (2,000 mg/2L, 4×10^{-3}M). Doxorubicin was eliminated from the treatment program. Patients were treated every 28 days. To date, 31 patients (28 with refractory ovarian carcinoma) have been treated with a total of 73 courses of this intraperitoneal chemotherapy regimen. Intravenous hydration and sodium thiosulfate were administered as previously described. Nephrotoxicity (serum creatinine >1.5 gm/dl), leukopenia (WBC <2,000/mm^3) and thrombocytopenia (platelets <75,000/mm^3) developed following 3%, 0%, and 5% of courses, respectively. Abdominal pain was mild in most patients, but several did require narcotic analgesia for 1-3 days following therapy. Eighteen of the 31 patients are presently evaluable for response to therapy. Nine (50%) have demonstrated objective responses including marked decrease or disappearance of ascites in six patients, conversion of positive cytology to negative in three patients and complete regression of enlarged retroperitoneal adenopathy in one patient. The activity of this regimen in patients with advanced refractory ovarian carcinoma appears comparable to the three-drug intraperitoneal combination, but with less local abdominal discomfort.

During our initial phase I trial of escalating dosages of intraperitoneal cisplatin with thiosulfate protection of the kidneys, we observed unexpected activity of this agent in malignant mesothelioma. While hematogenous dissemination is common with this tumor, the principle disease manifestations are generally confined to the primary site in the pleural or peritoneal cavities. Surgery and radiation therapy are of limited effectiveness in this tumor, and chemotherapy has only been demonstrated to be of marginal benefit (17). Cisplatin administered intravenously has been reported to produce objective responses in only 10% of patients treated, with the most active agent, doxorubicin, demonstrating activity in approximately 50% of patients with this disease (18).

To date, 11 patients (all male) with malignant mesothelioma have been treated with intracavitary cisplatin along with sodium thiosulfate on either an every three-week schedule or on a weekly schedule with three weekly cycles being followed by a three-week rest before the next course is started. With the weekly schedule, patients have received up to 270 mg/m^2 (90 mg/m^2/week x 3) every three weeks for a total of six courses. Toxicity, including bone marrow suppression, has been mild with no nephrotoxicity or local toxicity in the treated cavity being observed. Eight of the 11 patients demonstrated evidence of response, including one patient with peritoneal mesothelioma who attained a pathologically defined complete remission. Currently, patients with malignant mesothelioma receiving intracavitary cisplatin at our institution are treated with 100 mg/m^2 a week x 3 followed by a three-week rest. A total of six courses are administered. As malignant mesothelioma is an uncommon disease, it will take some time for us to accrue enough patients to define the activity and ultimate role of intracavitary cisplatin in the management of this disease.

As with tumors confined to the peritoneal cavity, malignant disease in the pleural cavity is ideally suited for direct intracavitary chemotherapy administration. Malignant pleural disease resulting in pleural effusions has classically been approached by instilling sclerosing agents in an effort to prevent fluid reaccumulation. Several chemotherapeutic agents, including bleomycin, nitrogen mustard and doxorubicin, have been used for this purpose. Unfortunately, this form of treatment requires chest tube drainage, results in considerable hospitalization time, is associated with significant and sometimes severe pain, and is only effective in approximately 50% of patients treated. In addition, the malignant tumor is usually not treated by this approach, with disease being free to progress locally and regionally.

With the demonstrated safety and efficacy of single-agent intracavitary chemotherapy and the potential *in vivo* synergy between cisplatin and cytarabine when present in the high concentrations attainable in the pleural cavity, we have recently instituted a trial of combination intrapleural chemotherapy. Seven previously heavily pretreated patients with pathologically documented malignant pleural disease have been treated with a total of 12 courses of an intrapleural regimen consisting of cisplatin (100 mg/m^2), cytarabine (60 mg, 10^{-3}M) and doxorubicin (3 mg, 18 μM) in a total treatment volume of 250 ml of normal saline. Sodium thiosulfate was simultaneously administered intravenously (4 gm/m^2 bolus, 12 g/m^2 infusion over 6 hours). Following drainage of as much pleural fluid as possible (through a percutaneously placed thoracentesis catheter), the treatment volume was administered.

Four hours later as much fluid as possible was removed. In patients receiving more than one treatment, therapy was repeated at 21 day intervals.

In the seven patients treated, there was no significant nephrotoxicity (serum creatinine >1.5 gm/dl), leukopenia (WBC <2,000/mm^3), or thrombocytopenia (platelet count <75,000/mm^3) following therapy. In addition, there were no complaints of pain during or following drug instillation. Nausea and vomiting were moderate in severity and reasonably well controlled with antiemetic agents. Two of seven patients (both with ovarian carcinoma) responded to treatment with dramatic subjective and objective improvement. Both patients demonstrated essentially complete disappearance of pleural fluid following the first treatment cycle and lasting five and seven months. The two responding patients eventually died of disease progression outside the chest; they never again experienced symptomatic difficulty with recurrent pleural effusions.

As in our intraperitoneal chemotherapy program, we have recently attempted to take further advantage of cisplatin/cytarabine concentration dependent synergy. Currently, we are treating patients with malignant pleural disease with cisplatin (100 mg/m^2) and a significantly escalated dosage of cytarabine (600 mg, 10^{-2}M) in a 250 ml treatment volume. To date, four patients (three refractory ovarian carcinoma, one adenocarcinoma of the lung) with malignant pleural effusions have been treated with this treatment regimen. All have demonstrated significant reductions in reaccumulation of pleural fluid. Again, there was no local pain, nephrotoxicity, or myelosuppression observed.

While it is possible the benefit we have demonstrated is due to a non-specific sclerosing effect of the therapy, we doubt this is the case for several reasons. First, sclerosing-agent therapy is commonly associated with significant pain. We have observed none. Second, we have made no attempt to assure tissue apposition between the parietal and visceral pleural surfaces, an important factor in the success of sclerosing therapy. Drainage is never complete in our patients and is only performed to attempt to allow maximum concentration of drugs in contact with tumor. Finally, several of the responding patients have actually had rapid fluid reaccumulation following therapy (demonstrated on chest x-ray), only to have the fluid disappear 2-3 weeks later. This suggests the effect of the therapy is not on the pleura directly but rather on the malignant cells themselves, and it is only when these cells are killed and removed that a clinical response will be observed.

Much work remains to be done in the area of cisplatin-based combination intracavitary chemotherapy. Optimal drugs and dosages, as well as appropriate scheduling, remain to be defined. Whether or not combination intracavitary chemotherapy will significantly improve survival of patients with malignant disease confined to body cavities must await carefully controlled clinical trials comparing this treatment approach to standard, systemically administered chemotherapy.

REFERENCES

1. Goldie JH, Coldman AJ: A mathematic model for relating the drug sensitivity of tumors to their spontaneous mutation rate. Cancer Treat Rep 63:1727-1733, 1979.
2. Dedrick RL, Myers CE, Bungay PM, DeVita VT Jr: Pharmacokinetic rationale for peritoneal drug administration in the treatment of ovarian cancer. Cancer Treat Rep 62:1-9, 1978.
3. Howell SB, Pfeifle CE, Wung WE, Olshen RA, Lucas WE, Yon JL, Green MR: Intraperitoneal cisplatin with systemic thiosulfate protection. Ann Intern Med 97:845-851, 1982.
4. Pfeifle CE, King ME, Howell SB: Pharmacokinetics and clinical efficacy of intraperitoneal cytarabine treatment of advanced ovarian cancer. Proc Am Soc Clin Oncol 2:150, 1983.
5. Ozols RF, Young RC, Speyer JL, Sugarbaker PH, Green R., Jenkins J, Myers CE: Phase I and pharmacological studies of adriamycin administered intraperitoneally to patients with ovarian cancer. Cancer 42:4265-4269, 1982.
6. Speyer JL, Collins JM, Dedrick RL, Brennan MF, Buckpitt AR, Londer H, DeVita VT Jr, Myers CE: Phase I pharmacological studies of 5-fluorouracil administered intraperitoneally. Cancer Res 40:567-572, 1980.
7. Pfeifle CE, Howell SB, Olshen RA, Wung WE: Intraperitoneal melphalan: A phase I study. Am Soc Clin Pharm Therap 33:223, 1983.
8. Howell SB, Chu BCF, Wung WE, Metha BM, Mendelsohn J: Long-duration intracavitary infusion of methotrexate with systemic leucovorin protection in patients with malignant effusions. J Clin Invest 67:1161-1170, 1981.
9. Jones RB, Collins JM, Myers CE, Brooks AS, Hubbard SM, Balow JE, Brennan MR, Dedrick RL, DeVita VT Jr: High-volume intraperitoneal chemotherapy with methotrexate in patients with cancer. Cancer Res 41:55-59, 1981.
10. Gyves J, Ensminger W, Niederhuber J, Manuzak P, Van Harken D, Janis MA, Stetson P, Knutsen C, Doan K: Phase I study of intraperitoneal (IP) 5 day continuous 5-FU infusion and bolus mitomycin C. Proc Am Soc Clin Oncol 1:15, 1982.

11. Katz ME, Schwartz PE, Kapp DS, Luikart S: Epithelial carcinoma of the ovary: current strategies. Ann Intern Med 95:98-111, 1981.
12. Williams CJ, Mead B, Arnold A, Green J, Buchanan R, Whitehouse M: Chemotherapy of advanced ovarian carcinoma: initial experience using a platinum-based combination. Cancer 49:1178-1783, 1982.
13. Cohen CJ, Goldberg JD, Holland JF, Bruckner HW, Deppe B, Gusberg SB, Wallach RC, Kabakow B, Rodin J: Improved therapy with cisplatin regimens for patients with ovarian carcinoma (FIGO stages III and IV) as measured by surgical end-staging (second-look operation). Am J Obstet Gynecol 145:955-967, 1983.
14. Wasserman TH, Comis RL, Goldsmith M, Handelsman H, Penta JS, Slavik M, Soper WP, Carter SK: Tabular analysis of the clinical chemotherapy of solid tumors. Cancer Chemother Rep 6(3):399-419, 1975.
15. Bergerat J-P, Green C, Drewinko B: Combination chemotherapy *in vitro*. IV. response of human colon carcinoma cells to combinations using cis-diamminedichloroplatinum. Cancer Biochem Biophy 3:173-180, 1979.
16. Bergerat J-P, Drewinko B, Corry P, Barlogie B, Ho DH: Synergistic lethal effect of cis-dichlorodiammineplatinum and 1-Beta-D-arabinofuranosylcytosine. Cancer Res 41:25-30, 1981.
17. Antman KH: Malignant mesothelioma. N Engl J Med 303:200-202, 1980.
18. Aisner J, Wiernik PH: Chemotherapy in the treatment of malignant mesothelioma. Sem Oncol 8:335-343, 1981.

INTRAVESICAL DOXORUBICIN FOR PROPHYLAXIS IN THE MANAGEMENT OF RECURRENT SUPERFICIAL BLADDER CARCINOMA - AN UPDATE

MARC B. GARNICK, BARBARA MAXWELL, ROBIN S. GIBBS, AND JEROME P. RICHIE

INTRODUCTION

The natural history of transitional cell carcinoma of the bladder that is superficial and limited to the mucosa or lamina propria is extremely variable. The 5-year survival rates range between 65 and 85 per cent. However, 50 to 70 per cent of the patients will have recurrent lesions of a similar or different stage or grade (1). In a detailed natural history study by the National Bladder Cancer Collaborative Group A, 30 per cent of the patients with stage T1 lesions (cancer limited to the lamina propria) had muscle invasion during a 3-year interval (2). Although the likelihood of muscle invasion was less than with stage Ta lesions (papillary noninvasive carcinoma), patients with poorly differentiated lesions eventually may have muscular invasion. Variables such as histopathologic findings, pathologic grade, anatomic location multiplicity of lesions, cytogenetic abnormalities of the exfoliated urothelial cells, presence of ABO surface antigens and the concomitant presence of cellular atypia or carcinoma *in situ* in surrounding areas are of prognostic importance when designing therapeutic strategies. The fact that traditional endoscopic resection and fulguration of these superficial lesions still are accompanied by a substantial number of recurrences underscores the need for additional therapy to decrease the number of recurrences, increase the duration between recurrences, decrease the likelihood of subsequent muscle, lymphatic and ultimately disseminated spread, and, hopefully, eradicate the disease.

Intravesical administration of antineoplastic agents is one option in the management of patients with superficial bladder cancer. The rationale underlying its use includes the elimination of multifocal microscopic foci of cancer and the elimination of pre-neoplastic and carcinoma *in situ* changes, two elements that are believed to be important in the pathogenesis of new and invasive lesions. Two additional considerations are achievement of high regional drug concentrations in the bladder mucosa and lamina propria and minimization of systemic toxicity by selection of agents that will have the least amount of absorption through the bladder wall.

We describe our updated experience in the prophylactic management of patients with multiple recurrent superficial bladder carcinoma with intravesical doxorubicin. This experience in 45 patients updates our previous study of 27 patients recently reported (3).

MATERIALS AND METHODS

Patients

Forty-four of 45 patients had multiple recurrent superficial stage O or A transitional carcinoma of the bladder or carcinoma *in situ*. One patient had early superficial muscular invasion. Patients who had recurrent disease while receiving intravesical thiotepa also were studied. There were 27 men and 18 women between 46 and 83 years of age (median age was 67 years). The mean duration of disease at entry was 5.5 years with a range of 3 months to 18 years. There were 7 patients who had disease greater than 5 years, and 15 patients who had received intravesical thiotepa were judged to have progressive disease while on this therapy. The staging systems used in this study were that of Jewett and Strong and the tumor, nodes, and metastasis systems of the International Union Against Cancer, in which disease was classified as being carcinoma *in situ* (Tis), stage O (Ta) with disease limited to the mucosa, and stage A (Tl) with disease limited to the lamina propria (4). Of the patients, 6 had carcinoma *in situ* only, 15 had stage O disease, 2 had stage O and carcinoma *in situ*, 18 had stage A, and 3 had stage A and carcinoma *in situ*. Eight patients had grade 1, 15 had grade 2, 16 had grade 3 lesions, and 6 had carcinoma _in situ_ only. Of the 45 patients, 15 had class 5 urinary tract cytology findings at the time of study initiation.

Study Design

Patients underwent cystoscopy and complete resection of all bladder tumors approximately 1 week before initiation of intravesical doxorubicin. It should be emphasized that all of our patients were rendered free of disease endoscopically (including the patient with superficial muscle invasion) before initiation of intravesical therapy. Intravesical doxorubicin was administered every 3 weeks for a total of 8 doses, then every 6 weeks for 2 doses, and then every 12 weeks for 2 doses. Therapy then ended for patients who were rendered free of disease. Thus, a total of 12 treatments was administered during 60 weeks from initiation of therapy. In addition, urinary tract cytology specimens were obtained from all patients. Pharmacologic analyses of peripheral blood samples for doxorubicin and adriamycinol levels were performed on the first 17 patients using high performance liquid chromatography methodology with a lower limit of detection of 10 ng./ml (5).

The starting dose was 60 mg. diluted in 40 to 50 ml. normal saline and was administered via a Foley catheter. Dwell time was 1 hour. Dose escalation after three treatments at one dose was extended through 70, 80, and 90 mg. The majority of patients received 70, 80, or 90 mg. per treatment. A total of 581 courses was administered to the 45 patients.

RESULTS

Toxicity

The side effects of intravesical therapy are shown in Table 1. Of the patients, 31 per cent had episodes of dysuria, 35.5 per cent had frequency, 35.5 per cent had hematuria, and 18 per cent had bladder spasms at some point during therapy. Two episodes of urinary tract infection developed early in the study. There seemed to be no clear-cut dose effect nor cumulative toxicity for dysuria or frequency.

Table 1. Toxicity of intravesical doxorubicin in 45 patients

	No. Pts. (N=45)	(%)	% Courses (N=581) 70 mg.	80 mg.	90 mg.
Dysuria	14	(31.1)	6	6	2
Frequency	16	(35.5)	12	10	15
Hematuria	16	(35.5)	4	8	3
Suprapubic discomfort	4	(8.8)	1	1	< 1
Urinary tract infection	2	(4.4)	1	0	< 1
Local irritation	5	(11.1)	0	2	2
Anaphylaxis	1	(2.2)			

Pharmacology

Plasma pharmacology was studied in 17 patients. Trace levels of doxorubicin were seen in only one patient with one drug course. Otherwise, doxorubicin plasma levels, if at all existent, were below the limit of sensitivity. Consistent with the lack of systemic absorption of doxorubicin, myelosuppression was not seen.

Therapeutic effectiveness

Of the 45 patients, 25 (55.5 per cent) have maintained complete remission status, with no evidence of any residual carcinoma detected endoscopically, and have had persistently negative urine cytology studies (Table 2). This group includes 10 patients who had become refractory to thiotepa. Of these 25 responding patients, 7 had stage O disease, 2 had stage O with carcinoma *in situ*, 14 had stage A disease, 1 had stage A disease with carcinoma *in situ*, and 1 had carcinoma *in situ* only (Table 3). Disease recurred in 17 patients (37.7 per cent), including 7 with invasive disease (Tables 4 and 5). Cystoscopy has remained grossly negative in 3 patients (6.6 per cent) who have had positive class 5 cytology studies. Of the 11 patients with carcinoma *in situ*, 2 patients had progressive disease, and 1 patient had persistently positive urinary cytology results. The median duration of follow up in the 45 patients is 16 months, with a range of 3 to 42 months (Table 2).

Table 2. Intravesical doxorubicin response rate and duration

	No./Total (%)
Complete response (no recurrence, neg. cytology)	25/45 (55.5)
Failure:	17/45 (37.7)
Recurrence without invasion to deeper layers	10/45 (22.2)
Recurrence with invasion to deeper layers	7/45 (15.5)
Persistent class 5 cytology, negative cystoscopy	3/45 (6.6)

Median duration of response was 16 months (range: 3-42 months)

Table 3. Grade and stage of complete responding patients* (N=25)

Stage	Grade 1	2	3
O (Ta)	4	2	3
A (T1)	2	7	6

*carcinoma *in situ* only = 1 patient

DISCUSSION

A variety of chemotherapeutic and immunotherapeutic agents administered intravesically has been found to be effective in definitive as well as prophylactic therapy of superficial bladder carcinoma. Included among such agents are thiotepa, mitomycin C, bacillus Calmette-Guerin and others (1). The most common form of intravesical therapy, thiotepa, is associated with systemic absorption, resulting in myelosuppression and thrombocytopenia. The use of doxorubicin, which seems not to undergo any systemic absorption when used in the present dose and schedule, offers an attractive alternative to the more standard therapies. Interestingly, recent evidence has indicated that doxorubicin can exert its cytotoxic activity without ever entering the cells. While the principal target was believed to be intercalation of deoxyribonucleic acid, the cytotoxic action of doxorubicin may involve interactions at the cell surface (6).

Dosage and schedule of intravesical therapy used in our

Table 4. Grade and stage of patients demonstrating recurrence without invasion* (N=10)

Stage	Grade 1	2	3
O (Ta)	2	3	0
A (T1)	0	2	1

*carcinoma *in situ* only = 2 patients

Table 5. Grade and stage of patients demonstrating recurrence with invasion* (N=7)

Stage	1	2	3
O (Ta)	0	0	2
A (T1)	0	0	2
B (T2)	0	1	0

*carcinoma *in situ* only = 2 patients

study were tolerated extremely well. Occasionally, irritative symptoms developed, which tended not to be cumulative and did not necessitate discontinuation of therapy in any patient. The only patient requiring therapy discontinuation following treatment with a 70 mg dose of doxorubicin demonstrated an anaphylactic reaction (hypotension, bronchospasm) on each of two separate occasions.

The need for multiple endoscopic tumor resections has been eliminated substantially in the majority of patients treated with this regional approach. Our results suggest that intravesical doxorubicin can serve as an effective agent to reduce or prevent recurrent bladder tumors in a high-risk population who have already demonstrated the proclivity for recurrent disease. The schedule of administration was tolerated extremely well, with no patient requiring drug discontinuation for local irritative problems. The search must continue to identify other active biological agents that may ultimately improve our current therapeutic results.

REFERENCES

1. Soloway MS: The management of superficial bladder cancer. Cancer (45): 1856-1865, 1980.
2. Heney NM, Ahmed S, Flanagan MJ, Frable W, Corder MP, Haferman MD, Hawkins IR: Superficial bladder cancer: progression and recurrence. J Urol (130):1083-1086, 1983.
3. Garnick MB, Schade D, Israel M, Maxwell B, Richie JP: Intravesical doxorubicin for prophylaxis in the management of recurrent superficial bladder carcinoma. J Urol (131): 43-46, 1984.
4. Prout GR Jr, Garnick MB, Canellos GP: The bladder. In: Holland JF, Frei E III (eds) Cancer Medicine. 2nd ed. Lea & Febiger, Philadelphia, 1982, pp. 1896-1912.
5. Israel M, Pegg WJ, Wilkinson PM, Garnick MB: Liquid chromatographic analysis of adriamycin and its metabolites in biological fluids. J Liquid Chromatog (1): 795-809, 1978.
6. Tritton TR, Yee G: The anticancer agent adriamycin can be actively cytotoxic without entering cells. Science (217): 248-250, 1982.

DEGRADABLE STARCH MICROSPHERES

WILLIAM D. ENSMINGER, PH.D., M.D.

INTRODUCTION

There is a need for new and more potent therapies against regionally confined tumors. The totally implanted pump has come into widespread usage, generating a large patient population where defined, repeated arterial access is possible. In most patients receiving hepatic arterial chemotherapy in particular, responses are not complete, and, thus, there is a need to add to our present armamentarium. As described elsewhere in this volume, as intra-arterial blood flow drops, the drug exposure for an agent infused into that artery rises in an inverse manner. Mechanisms for selectively decreasing regional intra-arterial flow can thus improve the regional drug exposure. Microparticulates, or microspheres of appropriate size given intra-arterially, represent one means to decrease blood flow through small nutrient arterioles and capillaries and, when combined with intra-arterial drugs, represent chemo-embolization therapy. Other studies described below suggest that, in the liver at least, tumors are hypervascular relative to surrounding liver, so that more microspheres selectively lodge in the tumor microcirculation. Although a variety of microparticulates are available, only one product, starch microspheres (Spherex, Pharmacia) has been developed to a stage where phase II efficacy testing has been initiated.

TUMOR MICROVASCULATURE AND BLOOD FLOW

Radiolabelled microparticulates in the form of Tc99m-macroaggregated albumin (TcMAA) have been extensively utilized intra-arterially as a means of mimicking drug-flow distribution at low infusion rates[1]. Observations made during hepatic artery perfusion scans (HAPS) with these (approximately 35 micron diameter) particles have provided insight into the functional microcirculation of hepatic tumors in patients.

The evoked new capillary bed generated by tumor growth generally develops at the periphery, so that the most vascularized area is at the outer rim of the tumor mass[2]. Although the central core of many tumor nodules in the liver is hypovascular, the periphery of the tumor nodule is generally hypervascular relative to normal liver, as demonstrated by TcMAA deposition during tomographic HAPS after hepatic arterial injection[3, 4]. The TcMAA deposition pattern on HAPS is consistent with the distribution of tumor cell viability and growth, the central core of the tumor often being necrotic and the peripheral rim of actively proliferating tumor cells having an excellent blood supply[2, 5]. The presence or absence of a hypovascular core appears to relate more to the size of the tumor nodule than to tumor type[4]. Nodules below 9 cm in diameter are uniformly hypervascular, whereas those over 9 cm in diameter display a hypovascular core and a hypervascular rim as ascertained by radionuclide tomographic angiography. The density of vessels in the hypervascular regions of tumor nodules appears to be 2- to 6-fold greater than in normal liver[4].

It is reasonable to assume that TcMAA deposition would be directly related to deposition of similarly sized (40 micron diameter) starch particles and that microregional intravascular blood volume relates as well to TcMAA deposition at the precapillary-arteriolar level. Thus, when microspheres of 40 micron diameter are injected as a homogenous suspension into the hepatic artery, they should lodge in the hepatic arterial microvasculature in direct proportion to varying blood flow throughout that watershed. The hepatic arterial injection of TcMAA (lung scanning agent) with nuclear tomography not only provides a means to determine the relative blood flow distribution between normal liver and tumor nodules within liver, but also to monitor selective delivery of therapeutic microspheres to tumor when TcMAA and therapeutic microspheres are admixed prior to intraarterial injection.

STARCH MICROSPHERES

Due to tumor hypervascularity, starch microspheres should lodge selectively in tumors and mimic the distribution pattern seen by radionuclide tomographic angiography with TcMAA, as described above. Depending directly upon the number of microspheres injected relative to the number of precapillary arterioles in the vascular bed infused, flow reduction will occur in a relative manner. At sufficiently high doses approximating 90 million biodegradable starch microspheres, hepatic arterial blood flow can be totally blocked in about 25% of patients [6, 7]. By 30 minutes after hepatic arterial injection, the starch microspheres are completely lysed by serum amylase and flow resumes through the hepatic arterial tree as ascertained by contrast angiograms. In the remaining 75% of patients, hepatic arterial flow decreases by 80% and arterial-venous shunting occurs[7]. As hepatic arterial flow is reduced, the advantage of an arterial infusion will increase in an inversely proportional manner.

A number of phase I investigative studies using chemotherapeutic drugs with biodegradable starch microspheres have been performed over the past several years[7-10]. The concurrent hepatic arterial injection of a suspension of starch microspheres in a drug solution has the potential of temporarily holding the drug solution in the hepatic arterial microcirculatory bed, thus allowing more time for the higher drug concentration to move into surrounding tissue. Bischlorethylnitrosourea (BCNU) and mitomycin C have been examined in conjunction with starch microspheres given via the hepatic artery [7,9]. These agents were chosen due to their rapid tissue uptake and mechanism of action as alkylating agents (i.e., peak drug levels are usually important determinants of cytotoxic effect). In addition, mitomycin may be activated (bioreduced) more highly in ischemic regions where microspheres have blocked blood flow[11]. Due to increased drug delivery to the liver and hepatic tumor, systemic drug exposure is reduced up to 90% for BCNU and 60% for mitomycin C when drug is given with starch microspheres as compared to drug injection alone[7, 9]. Based upon the decreased systemic drug deposition, drug delivery to the liver should be increased an additional 5 to 10-fold when drug is given concurrently with starch microspheres. In hypervascular regions of tumors, more drug solution should be held up as compared to drug entrapment in the less vascular regions of normal liver. As the microspheres are digested, their diameter progressively decreases (from 40 μm initially), and the drug column moves distally into the capillary bed. Due to complete dissolution of the starch microspheres by 30 minutes post-injection, subsequent doses can be administered without destroying access to the tumor microcirculation.

As the dose of starch microspheres injected is increased, progressive extrahepatic shunting of microspheres often occurs. This will work against the regional selectivity one is trying to achieve[10]. For example, the average amount of microspheres shunted to the lungs is 15% with 6 million microspheres and rises progressively to 27% when 90 million microspheres are injected (Table 1)[10]. As the number of starch microspheres is increased, symptoms such as epigastric burning and right upper quadrant discomfort progressively increase in frequency and severity (Table 1). It appears that 36 million microspheres (a 6 ml suspension of the standard formulation) are well tolerated and achieve at least 80% of the effect (i.e., decreased systemic drug exposure) achieved with the highest dose tested, 90 million microspheres (Table 1)[9].

At the appropriate dose of 36 million (6 ml), starch microspheres are generally well tolerated. It is crucial, however, that a HAPS be performed with an admixture of TcMAA and the starch microspheres (6 ml) prior to drug therapy. In some patients, blood flow redistribution (either due to ischemia or actual microvasculatory blockade) occurs, so that microspheres go to the duodenum or stomach. Any flow to the stomach or duodenum when starch microspheres are given with drug will induce severe pain and can result in a non-healing erosive gastritis.

Other toxicities include the development of acute dyspnea if shunting of starch microspheres to the lung is 40% or more.

The abdominal discomfort (see above and Table 1) and (when it occurs) the dyspnea resolve in 10-15 minutes as the starch microspheres are digested by serum amylase. Potential toxicities which are seen with hepatic arterial infusion of drug alone and which may be potentiated by starch microspheres include vasculitis and sclerosing cholangitis. These latter toxicities, should they occur, may not be reversible.

Table 1. Comparison of 36 Million With 90 Million Starch Microspheres Given Into the Hepatic Artery

	Dosage Used	
	36 Million	90 Million
1. Reduction Systemic Exposure		
a. For BCNU	N.D.	70-90%
b. For Mitomycin	38%	44%
2. Lung Shunting	15±8%	27±10%
3. Abdominal Discomfort		
Mild-Moderate	25% of patients	40% of patients
Severe	5% of patients	50% of patients

CONCLUSION

Factors important to the safe use of starch microspheres have been defined. A reasonably appropriate dose of starch microspheres for administration concurrently with mitomycin, BCNU, or other drugs into the hepatic artery is 36 million particles or 6 ml of the formulated suspension (6 million/ml). Phase II studies using this dose of microspheres with mitomycin and BCNU into the hepatic artery in patients with measurable hepatic tumors have recently been initiated. Ultimately, a randomized phase III study comparing the efficacy of hepatic arterial drug (BCNU or mitomycin) alone versus drug with starch microspheres must be conducted.

REFERENCES

1. Kaplan WD, Ensminger WD, Come SE, Smith EH, D'Orsi CJ, Levin DC, Takvorian RW, Steele GD, Jr: Radionuclide angiography to predict patient response to hepatic artery chemotherapy. Cancer Treat Rep (64):1217-1222, 1980.
2. Warren BA: The vascular morphology of tumors. In: Peterson, HI (ed) Tumor blood circulation: Angiogenesis, vascular morphology and blood flow of experimental and human tumors. CRC Press, Inc., Florida, 1979, pp 1-47.
3. Gyves J, Ensminger W, Yang P, Thrall J, Cho K: Clinical utility of microspheres to assess and attack hepatic tumor microcirculation. Clin Res (30):418A, 1982.
4. Gyves J, Ensminger W, Thrall J, Cho K, Walker S: Dependence of hepatic tumor vascularity on tumor size. Clin Res (30):747A, 1982.
5. Ackerman NB, Heckmer PA: The blood supply of experimental liver metastases. V. Increased tumor perfusion with epinephrine. Am J Surg (140):625-631, 1980.
6. Aronsen KF, Hellenkant C, Holmberg J, Rothman U, Teder H: Controlled blocking of hepatic artery flow with enzymatically degradable microspheres combined with oncolytic drugs. Eur Surg Res (11):99-106, 1979.
7. Dakhil S, Ensminger W, Cho K, Niederhuber J, Doan K, Wheeler R: Improved regional selectivity of hepatic arterial BCNU with degradable microspheres. Cancer (50):631-635, 1982.
8. Lindell B, Aronsen KF, Nosslin B, Rothman ULF: Studies in pharmacokinetics and tolerance of substance temporarily retained in the liver by microsphere embolization. Ann Surg (187):95-99, 1978.

9. Gyves JW, Ensminger WD, VanHarken D, Niederhuber J, Stetson P, Walker S: Improved regional selectivity of hepatic arterial mitomycin by starch microspheres. Clin Pharmacol Therap (34):259-265, 1983.
10. Ziessman HA, Thrall JH, Gyves JW, Ensminger WD, Niederhuber JE, Tuscan M, Walker S: Quantitative hepatic arterial perfusion scintigraphy and starch microsphere in cancer chemotherapy. J Nucl Med (24):871-875, 1983.
11. Kennedy K, Rockwell S, Sartorelli A: Preferential activation of mitomycin C to cytotoxic metabolites by hypoxic tumor cells. Cancer Res (40):2356-2360, 1980.

MAGNETIC DRUG-CONTAINING MICROSPHERES*

R.C. RICHARDSON[1], G.S. ELLIOTT[1], J.M. BARTLETT[1], W.E. BLEVINS[1], W. JANAS[1], J.R. HALE[2], R.L. SILVER[3]

INTRODUCTION

Targeting of magnetic drug-containing microspheres is one of several regional/site-specific forms of chemotherapy evaluated in recent years. This article reviews the history of magnetic microspheres, including some laboratory-animal models used to evaluate such microspheres. It describes methods of vascular access using spontaneously occurring large-animal (canine) extremity tumors. It further describes a pilot study of such canine tumors when they are influenced by an externally placed electromagnet to localize magnetic human albumin microspheres containing doxorubicin.

HISTORY

In 1963 Meyers et al.(1) reported the feasibility of localizing micronized iron, 1-3 in diameter, at specific sites within dogs and rodents by using externally placed magnets. They used ^{59}Fe to demonstrate in situ entrapment of particles at the magnet site as well as the fate of the particles following one hour of magnetic entrapment. Standard radiographic and histologic techniques were used to visualize the iron particles. The particles could be stopped and seen radiographically in accessible veins, arteries, and other accessible organs, such as the esophagus. Distribution studies of radio-labeled particles showed that any micronized iron escaping the magnet site was transported to the liver, spleen, and lungs where it was trapped by reticuloendothelial tissue. The radioactivity associated with the iron particles that were initially

---

*This work was supported by the Purdue Comparative Oncology Program, Purdue School of Veterinary Medicine's Medical Illustration Department, and a grant from Eli Lilly and Company.

1. Purdue Comparative Oncology Program, Purdue University, West Lafayette, IN 47907

2. Francis Bitter National Magnet Laboratory, Massachusetts Institute of Technology, Cambridge, MA 02139

3. Michael Reese Hospital and Medical Center, Chicago, IL 60616

deposited at the magnet site slowly decreased over two weeks. It increased in the liver, spleen, and lungs over one week, and then slowly decreased in those organs. Microscopic studies confirmed the presence of iron particles in the liver, spleen, and lungs as well as in the glomeruli of the kidneys. Numerous particles were seen between the vessels and muscle bundles near the magnet site following one hour of continuous magnetic control. This article in 1963 was the first to suggest magnetically controlled iron particles as vehicles for carrying chemotherapeutic agents.

Fifteen years after the suggestion of Meyers et al.(1), Widder et al.(2) first described magnetic microspheres carrying water-soluble chemotherapeutic drugs. They hoped that the novel carrier system might prove to be an efficient method of obtaining high local drug concentrations and potentially decreasing unwanted side effects from unrestricted systemic circulation of chemotherapeutic agents. Magnetite (Fe_3O_4) was combined with human albumin through a water-in-oil emulsion polymerization to create magnetically responsive microspheres. Such spheres were magnetically influenced because of the Fe_3O_4 and were more resistant than micronized iron to magnetic clumping because the magnetizable material was coated with albumin, which created a charged particle. Magnetic clumping is an undesired feature since it prevents the spheres from being homogeneously distributed at the capillary level and causes them to form emboli which may infarct portions of the target circulation. The spheres described by Widder et al. were small enough to prevent the formation of microemboli. Such spheres were also biodegradable, minimally reactive with blood components, and non-toxic. Furthermore, they could accommodate a wide variety of water-soluble drugs.

Widder et al. used female retired breeder Sprague-Dawley rats. The ventral caudal artery was partially exposed at the base of the tail, and doxorubicin-bearing spheres (0.05 mg doxorubicin/kg) were infused under the influence of a permanent bipolar magnet. Following infusion, the catheter was removed, and the magnet was left in position for 30 minutes. After the 30 minute magnet time, one group of rats was sacrificed and examined for distribution of spheres within the tail. Another group was sacrificed 24 hours after the magnet was turned off and then examined for biodistribution of the microspheres. A third group of rats received doxorubicin-bearing microspheres without the influence of the magnet, while a fourth group received free doxorubicin via catheter into the ventral caudal artery (0.05 mg/kg) or femoral vein (5.0 mg/kg). Tissue distribution was determined by radiotracer techniques with ^{125}I-labeled microspheres as well as by electron microscopy

Drug concentration in different tissues was measured. Results showed that 1)approximately 50% of delivered spheres were trapped in the area of the magnet with no significant washout after the magnet was turned off; 2)doxorubicin from the spheres was detected only in the area directly under the magnet; 3)infusion of free doxorubicin via the ventral caudal artery at 0.05 mg/kg resulted in no detectable doxorubicin in the tail; 4)infusion of 5.0 mg/kg free doxorubicin via the femoral vein resulted in tissue levels equivalent to the microsphere-delivered drug; and 5)spheres not entrapped in the tail were found in the liver, spleen, and lungs, but significant (toxic) tissue levels of doxorubicin were not found in those organs. Entrapment without substantial washout, measured 24 hours after release of direct magnetic influence, suggested that the microspheres might be lodged in the vascular endothelium or might possibly have traversed the vascular basement membrane into interstitial tissues. The authors also inferred that partial thrombosis due to conglutination of the microspheres might have been responsible for the continued retention of the spheres. Electron microscopic evaluation of the skin directly under the magnet yielded results suggesting vascular exit, since microspheres were seen in and between endothelial cells. These observations provided impetus to test drug-bearing microspheres in experimental tumor models.

ANIMAL MODELING

Methods of Vascular Access for Microsphere Delivery to Tumors

A review of the literature demonstrates that intra-arterial access to extremities (e.g. limbs, tail) has been used more than any other route to deliver microspheres to tumors. Selective arterial catheterization may also be used to access hepatic, renal, pulmonary, pelvic, and head/neck sites of neoplasia. We have described methods of vascular access for delivery of microspheres to distal extremity tumors in dogs(3) and suggested that such a model makes an excellent comparison for extremity tumors of man. The purpose of our preliminary studies was to determine the usefulness of the tumor-bearing dog as a large-animal model before targeted drug delivery is attempted in humans. The similarities between spontaneous dog and human neoplasms include histopathologic type, cell kinetics, tumor volume and biologic behavior(4,5). In addition, dogs are closer to humans in size than are other animal models such as rodents. Size is of particular importance in vascular access to and magnetic influence across a neoplasm. Therefore, the size of the dog and the size of the tumor in relationship to the host make such an experimental system appropriate for our pre-clinical trials before Phase I trials in man are attempted. We used three vascular routes (intravenous, intra-arterial, and intramedullary) to evaluate spontaneous distal extremity tumors in dogs before infusing 1-3 magnetic microspheres. Vascular access was studied in the normal canine limb, in animals bearing soft-tissue sarcomas and in animals with osteogenic sarcomas.

Intravenous (IV) access to the tumors was accomplished by placing a tourniquet proximal to the tumor and installing a venous catheter in a retrograde manner (against the normal flow) in a vein draining the tumor. Contrast material was then infused into the tourniqueted vascular bed, forcing the media through venous-arterial shunts in the tumor. This demonstrated access to superficial, large-diameter vessels rather than to deep, small-diameter tumor vessels (Figures 1 and 2).

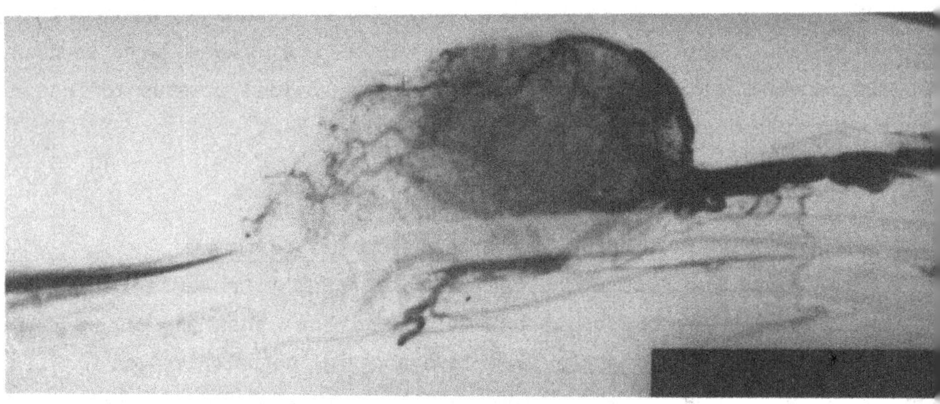

FIGURE 1. Angiogram showing retrograde intravenous filling of a non-osseous tumor (hemangiopericytoma) on the distal foreleg of a dog. Large-diameter vessels are visualized shunting around and through the tumor.

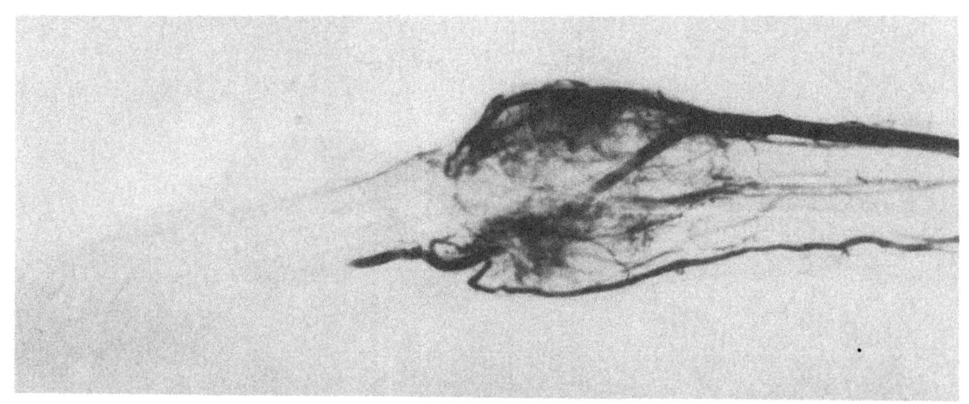

IGURE 2. Angiogram showing retrograde intravenous filling of a canine steogenic sarcoma affecting the distal radius. Contrast material has shunted rom the venous side of the tumor, across large-diameter vessels, and has illed an artery descending the posterior aspect of the foreleg. Neither the entral portion of the tumor nor vessels distal to the tumor are filled with ontrast material.

Intra-arterial (IA) contrast studies were accomplished by placing atheters in femoral arteries (via a carotid artery) for rear-limb tumors or in rachial arteries (via a femoral artery) for forelimb tumors. Uniform erfusion of tumor parenchyma was demonstrated for all extra-osseous tumors Figure 3). In bone tumors, osseous tissue was inconsistently perfused (Figure).

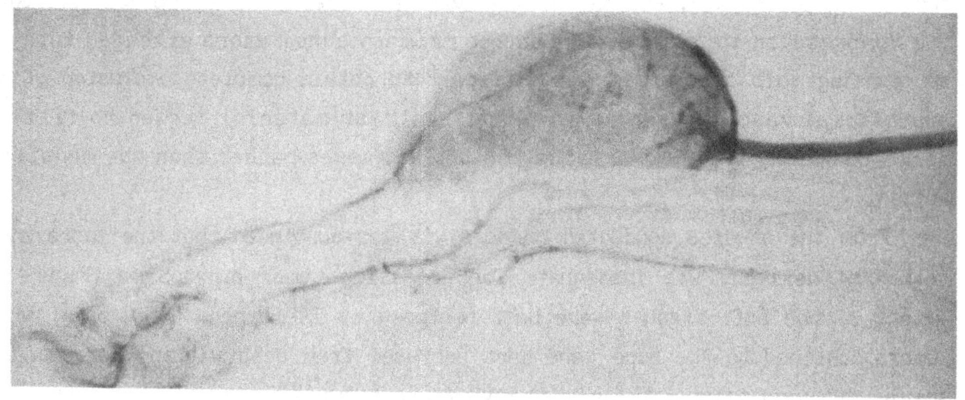

IGURE 3. Intra-arterial angiogram of a canine hemangiopericytoma. Contrast aterial has filled the small-diameter vessels throughout the mass as evidenced y the homogeneous distribution. The same tumor as in Figure 1 is evaluated.

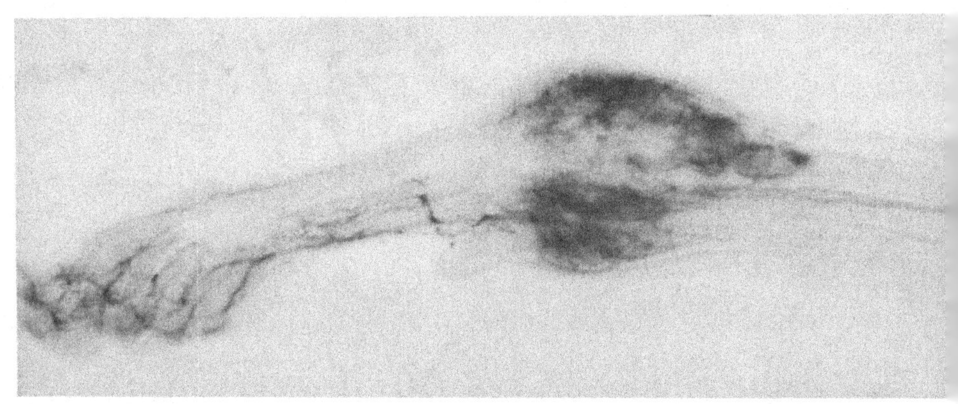

FIGURE 4. Intra-arterial angiogram of a canine osteogenic sarcoma. The extra-osseous tissues are well perfused, however the bony center fails to demonstrate perfusion. The same tumor as in Figure 2 is evaluated.

Intramedullary (IM) access to primary bone tumors was accomplished by placing a superficial venous catheter in a vein distal to the tumor. The limb was then wrapped in a whole-limb compression (Esmarch) tourniquet, thereby occluding all superficial arterial and venous blood-flow. Contrast material was then injected via an infusion pump into the catheter, forcing the injected material into deep (intramedullary) vascular channels rather than through the normal venous routes (Figure 5). Contrast material traversed the medullary space, exiting at the next proximal joint space not covered by the compression tourniquet. When the primary bone tumors extended into the surrounding soft tissue, it was difficult to obtain complete occlusion of the superficial vasculature; as a result, contrast material tended to fill the large-diameter veins overlying the tumor masses rather than the medullary spaces.

From the studies conducted on dogs, it was concluded that the intravenous method of delivery was inadequate for accessing tumor parenchyma (Figure 6). Tumors of the soft tissues were best perfused by IA methods (Figure 7), while tumors confined to the bone were best perfused from deep within the medullary space, outward toward the periphery of the tumor (Figure 8). If a tumor is comprised of both osseous and extra-osseous components, a combined IA and IM technique appears to be necessary to perfuse the neoplasm completely (Figure 9).

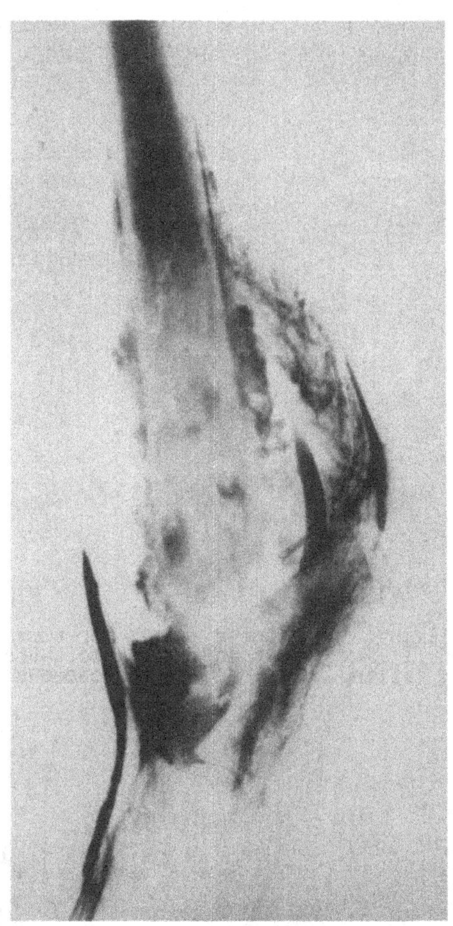

FIGURE 5. Intramedullary contrast study of a canine osteogenic sarcoma of the distal tibia. Contrast material has entered the medullary space and can be seen filling the medullary canal. A few large-diameter veins that were not occluded by the compression bandage are observed on the posterior aspect of the tumor.

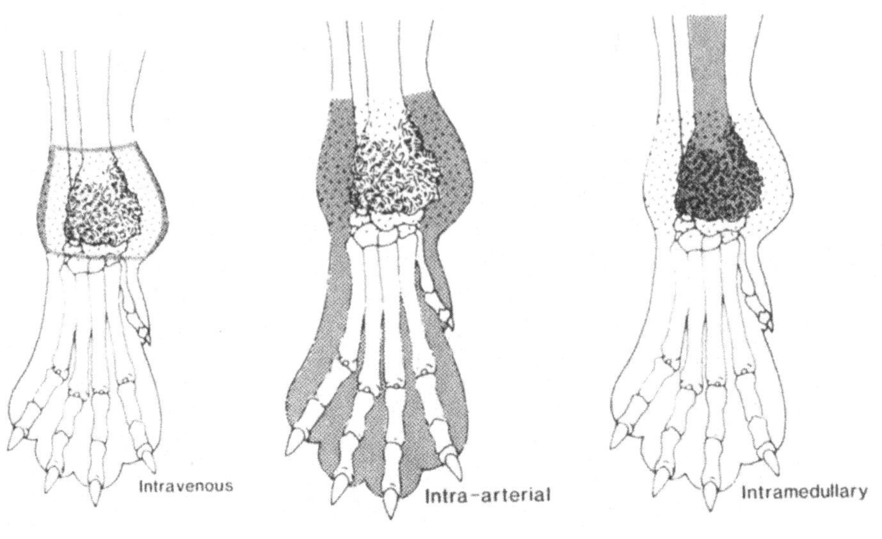

FIGURE 6 FIGURE 7 FIGURE 8

FIGURE 6. Intravenous filling. Inadequate access for tumor delivery.
FIGURE 7. Intra-arterial filling. Best access for soft-tissue tumors.
FIGURE 8. Intramedullary filling. Best access for osseous tumors.

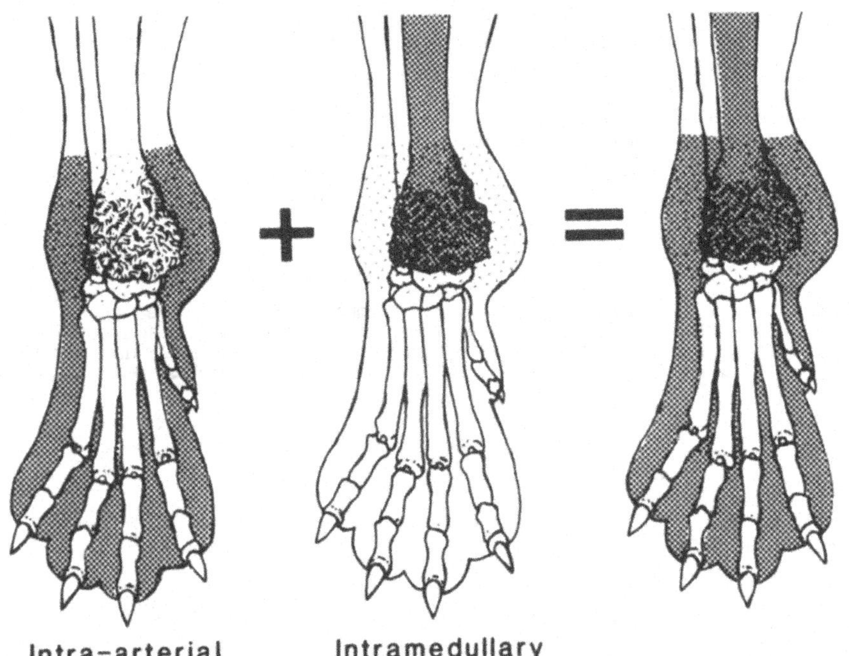

FIGURE 9. Intra-arterial/intra-medullary filling. Best access for combined soft-tissue/osseous tumors.

Localization of Magnetic Microspheres in Canine Osteogenic Sarcomas

We have described the use of ^{99m}Tc to label magnetically responsive human albumin microspheres to follow their fate after IV, IA, and IM delivery to the extremities of 36 dogs with spontaneously occurring osteogenic sarcomas(6). The spheres were infused while the target site was exposed to an external magnetic field created by a 5-kW electromagnet prepared at the Francis Bitter National Magnet Laboratory, Cambridge, MA. The single pole of this magnet had a 10-cm chisel-shaped tip that could be freely moved in all directions to facilitate external positioning over the tumor. Once the magnet was in position, power was applied and infusion of the labeled microspheres was begun. The tumor site was maintained under magnetic influence for 30 minutes post-infusion, and then the power to the magnet was turned off. Redistribution of the labeled spheres from the tumor to the rest of the body was monitored by an external gamma-counting device (crystal scintillation detector).

Survival Studies--Tumor localization of the radio-labled microspheres was evaluated using two separate criteria. The first criterion was a measure of the permanence of localization once the magnetic influence had been terminated and was determined by monitoring the retention of radioactivity at the target site as a function of time after the treatment. Data were collected for 15 minutes beginning at the time that the magnetic influence was removed. Generally, the radioactive counts stabilized within the 15-minute counting period, thus suggesting that redistribution of the radio-labeled spheres from the target site was essentially complete. These data were reported as the retention value, which is the ratio of the count rate at the end of the monitoring period to the count rate at the start of the period.

The second criterion was a relative evaluation of the biodistribution of the radio-labled spheres between the target site and the lungs and liver. A tumor index value was generated by dividing the tumor count by the sum of the counts over the tumor, the lungs, and the liver. Admittedly, the tumor index is a relative indicator of biodistribution and does not take into consideration either the total activity administered or any differences in counting geometries from dog to dog; however, when both the retention value and the tumor index are determined for a number of studies, they could indicate how efficiently different routes of administration carry and localize microspheres.

Intravenous infusion was studied with and without the influence of the magnetic field. Without the magnet, the retention of the radio-labeled spheres at the target site ranged from 67-98% after the tourniquet was released. The tumor index ranged from 0.49-0.96. When the magnet was used, retention ranged from 73-99%, and the tumor index ranged from 0.40-0.86. No difference could be discerned between the group that was infused with the tumor under the magnetic influence and the group infused without the magnet.

Intra-arterial infusion was also evaluated with and without magnetic influence. Without magnetic localization, retention in evaluable animals ranged from 25-65%, and the tumor index ranged from 0.40-0.44. When the magnet was used, retention ranged from 84-97%, and the tumor index ranged from 0.05-0.91. Magnetic influence, therefore, seems to cause a definite improvement in tumor retention.

Intramedullary infusion revealed a retention of 79-96% and a tumor index of 0.27-0.38 in typical tumors infused without the magnetic influence. A 48-96% retention of radio-labeled spheres and a tumor index of 0.07-0.70 was seen when the magnet was used. As in the intravenous infusion, there seemed to be little difference in the retention values caused by the magnet.

Sacrifice Studies--Twelve of the dogs were sacrificed immediately after infusion. In nine of them the tumor was removed, cross-sectioned, and evaluated by either rectilinear scanning or gamma scintigraphy to locate the labeled spheres within the tumor. Radiographs of the tumor sections were also made to evaluate osseous vs. extra-osseous tumor. One additional dog served as a control for sphere distribution and received the labeled spheres in a normal intravenous manner. Eight dogs were sacrificed following intra-arterial studies, and three after intramedullary perfusion. All dogs underwent complete necropsies to collect tissues for radionuclide studies. As expected, the primary biodistribution of the radio-labeled spheres outside the tumor was in the lungs, liver, spleen, and kidneys. The most striking observations of the sacrifice studies came from evaluating tumor sections by either rectilinear scanning or gamma scintigraphy. Intra-arterial administration of spheres very clearly filled only the soft-tissue components of the tumor (Figures 10-13), while intramedullary administration selectively filled the osseous portions (Figures 14 and 15). The magnet had a clear-cut influence on localizing radio-labeled spheres administered intra-arterially, while such influence was not as obvious in the intramedullary method. Angiographic studies had precisely predicted microsphere delivery and localization. It became apparent in this pilot study that appropriate angiography should precede any attempts to deliver microspheres to tumors, thereby assuring adequate access to the desired sites.

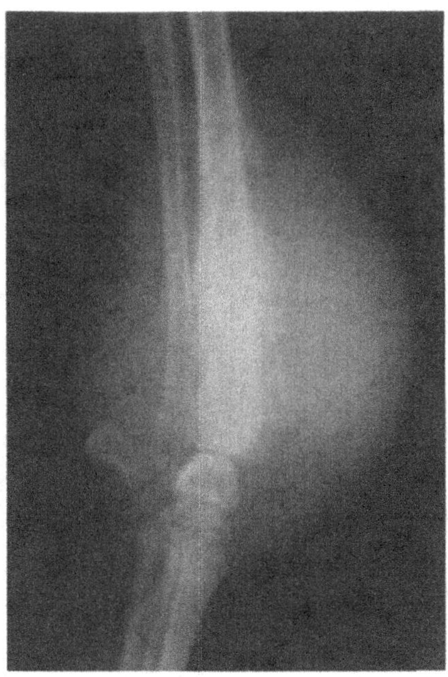

IGURE 10. Radiograph of the distal forelimb of a dog with osteogenic sarcoma. he tumor demonstrates a large amount of soft-tissue invasion.

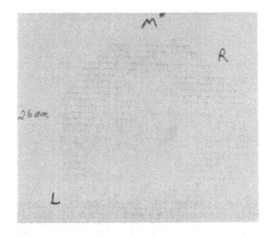

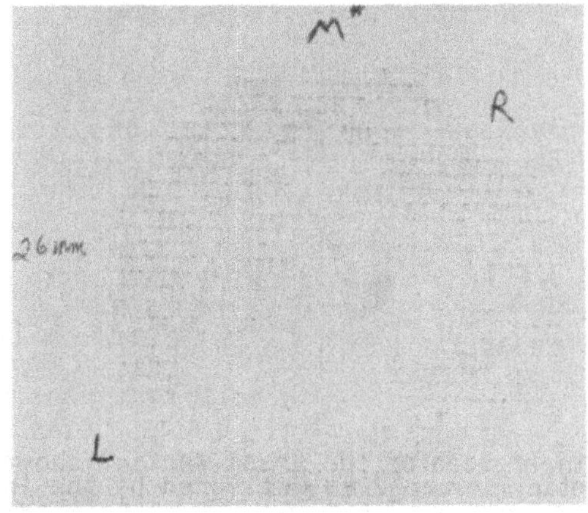

IGURE 11. Rectilinear scan of a cross-section from the tumor shown in Figure 0 using ^{99m}Tc-labelled magnetic microspheres following intra-arterial nfusion. Preferential delivery to the extra-osseous portions is present. he magnet has caused localization within the tissues closest to the pole ip. The magnet placement is marked with the letter "M".

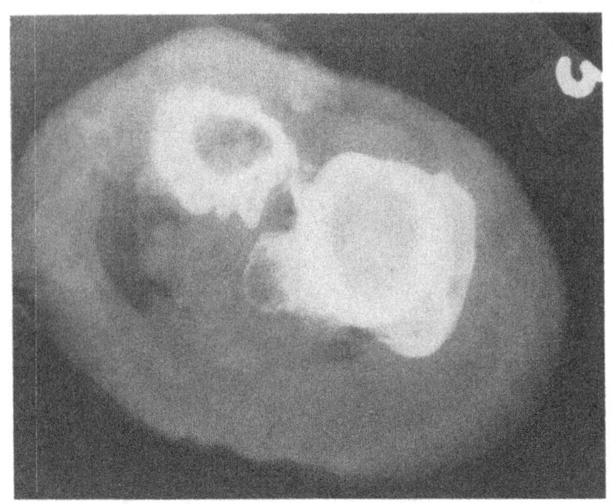

FIGURE 12. Radiograph of a cross-section of a canine osteogenic sarcoma with extension into the surrounding tissues.

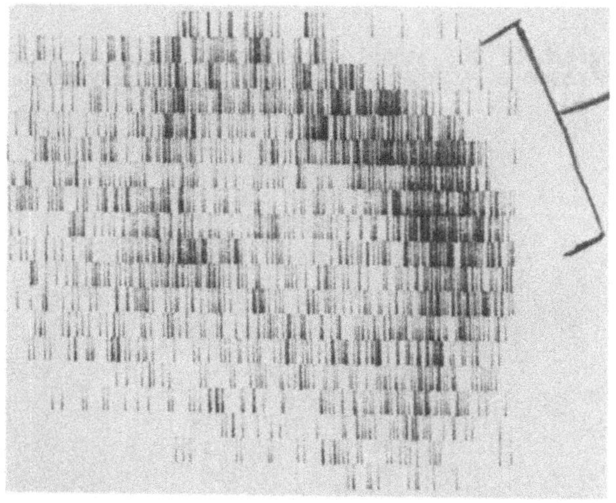

FIGURE 13. Rectilinear scan of the cross-section shown in Figure 12 using ^{99m}Tc-labelled magnetic microspheres delivered by the intra-arterial route. The soft tissues are best perfused and the magnet has caused the greatest holding immediately beneath the pole tip. Magnet placement is marked with a heavy bar.

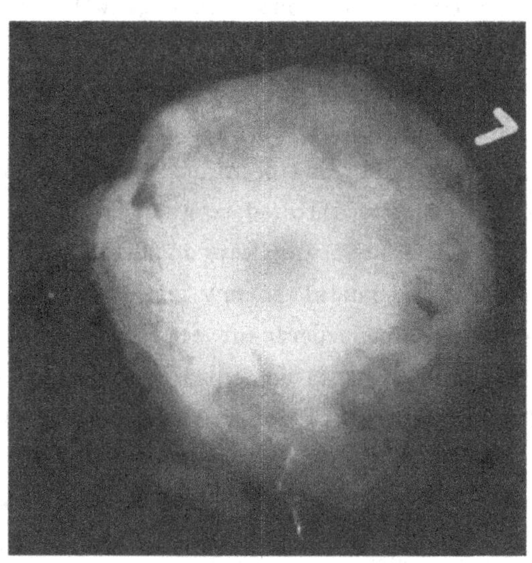

FIGURE 14. Radiograph of a cross-section of a canine osteogenic sarcoma.

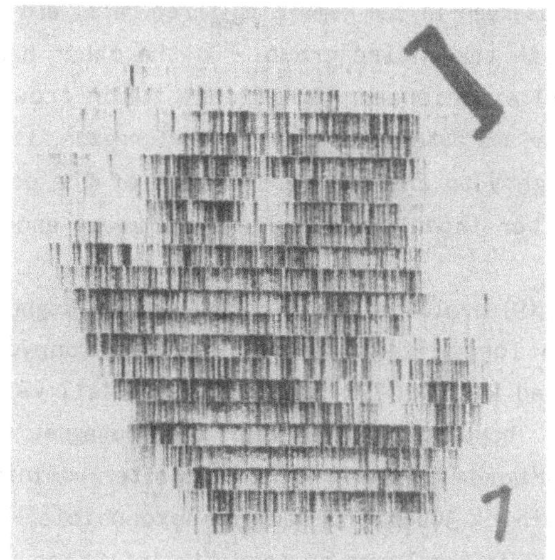

FIGURE 15. Rectilinear scan of the cross-section shown in Figure 14 using ^{99m}Tc-labelled magnetic microspheres following intramedullary infusion. The bony portions of the tumor are selectively filled. Minimal lateralization of the spheres has occurred secondary to magnet placement. The heavy bar marks magnet placement.

Tumor Response

Response to therapy using induced tumors in rodent models was described by Widder et al.(7, 8), Sugibayashi et al.(9), and Morris et al.(10). Rats bearing either Yoshida sarcoma tail implants or AH 7974 lung metastases were used. Therapeutic response to magnetic drug-containing microspheres has not been reported in animals with spontaneously occurring neoplasia. Our preliminary findings describe such responses in dogs with naturally occurring osteogenic sarcomas of the extremities.

Widder et al.(7, 8) described a dramatic tumor remission in rats bearing Yoshida sarcomas after being treated by targeted magnetic albumin microspheres containing doxorubicin. Tumor cells had been inoculated subcutaneously in the tails of rats, and the tumors were allowed to grow to an average size of 1 X 4.5 cm before treatment. Drug-bearing microspheres were infused intra-arterially through the ventral caudal artery and localized by a permanent magnet placed over the tumor. The experiment compared the response of tumors in rats receiving magnetically influenced drug-bearing spheres (0.5 mg doxorubicin per kg of body weight) to controls receiving IV doxorubicin (5 mg/kg), IA doxorubicin (5 and 0.5 mg/kg), placebo spheres with magnetic holding, or drug-bearing spheres (0.5 mg doxorubicin per kg body weight) without magnetic holding. Of the 12 rats treated in the experimental group, 9 demonstrated complete remission of their tumors after a single dose. Marked tumor regression was observed in the remaining three rats, and no metastases or deaths were observed in the entire group. On the other hand, all control groups (10 rats/group) experienced significant tumor growth with 80-100% demonstrating widespread metastasis to the inguinal region, liver, kidneys, lungs, and heart. Eighty to one hundred percent of the control rats died between 13-16 days after inoculation. The experiment ended 29 days after treatment.

Sugibayashi et al.(9) evaluated doxorubicin-bearing magnetic microspheres in rats with AH 7974 lung metastases. They used Donryu rats that had previously been infused with AH 7974 cells via the tail veins, causing the pulmonary metastases. They applied a bipolar electromagnet over the sternum and back of the rats. Magnet time was 10 minutes after administration of 5 mg of microspheres containing 300 micrograms of doxorubicin. The plan was to concentrate the spheres in the lungs by magnetic influence. They used radio-labeled spheres to demonstrate a 2-fold increase of microspheres in the lung when magnetic influence was present compared to studies conducted without the magnet. Even though significant numbers of microspheres did lodge in the liver, spleen, and heart when the magnet was in place, the numbers were even greater when no magnetic influence was present. An 8-fold increase of doxorubicin was obtained in the lungs with the magnetically influenced microspheres when compared with an equivalent dosage of free drug. Histopathologic examination of lung tissue showed that rats treated with microspheres demonstrated greater antitumor effects than did those treated with free drug. Increases in lung weights caused by tumor did not occur as rapidly in the microsphere-treated group as they did in either the free drug or untreated groups. Finally, mean survival times of the group treated with magnetically localized, drug-bearing microspheres were significantly longer than in either of the other groups.

Morris et al.(10) reported that magnetically responsive albumin microspheres containing vindesine sulfate caused complete remission in 75% of rats with Yoshida sarcomas implanted in their tails. The animals which did not demonstrate complete remission showed marked tumor regression, for an overall regression rate of 95%. No metastases were observed in the treatment group. Control groups were either untreated or treated with free vindesine sulfate or vindesine sulfate spheres without magnetic localization; 90-100% of the control animals demonstrated tumor growth, metastases, and death. The study was similar to that of Widder et al.(7, 8). Drug-bearing magnetic microspheres at dosages of 0.5 or 2.5 mg/kg were used.

In studies done in the Purdue Comparative Oncology Program, we have administered doxorubicin-bearing magnetic microspheres to 27 dogs with spontaneously occurring osteogenic sarcomas. Four demonstrated a measurable 50%) decrease in tumor size as evaluated by radiographic and clinical methods. Three more dogs demonstrated subjective improvement by resolution of clinical signs (e.g. lameness, pain). Therapeutic response was observed when ^{99m}Tc-labeled human albumin microspheres bearing doxorubicin were used to evaluate vascular access, sphere distribution, and magnetic influence in the studies previously described(3,6). All responding dogs developed recurrent tumor or relapse of clinical signs 6-12 weeks following therapy. Eight of the dogs received drug-bearing spheres by the intravenous route, eight by the intramedullary route and eleven by the intra-arterial route. No dogs in the intravenous administration group were observed to have a therapeutic response; three dogs in the intra-arterial group demonstrated partial remission based on tumor measurements and radiographic re-ossification of lytic lesions (Figures 16 and 17); and one dog in the intramedullary group showed remission of clinical and radiographic signs (Figures 18 and 19).

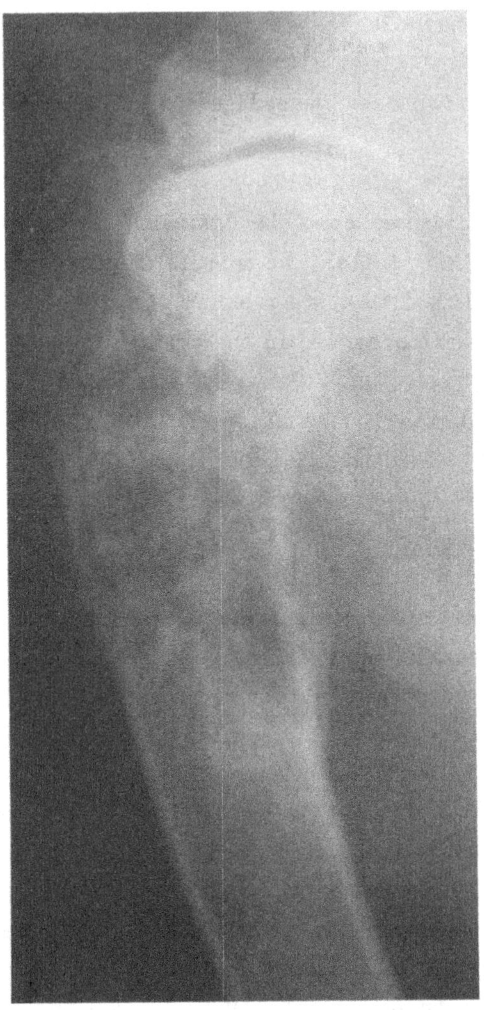

FIGURE 16

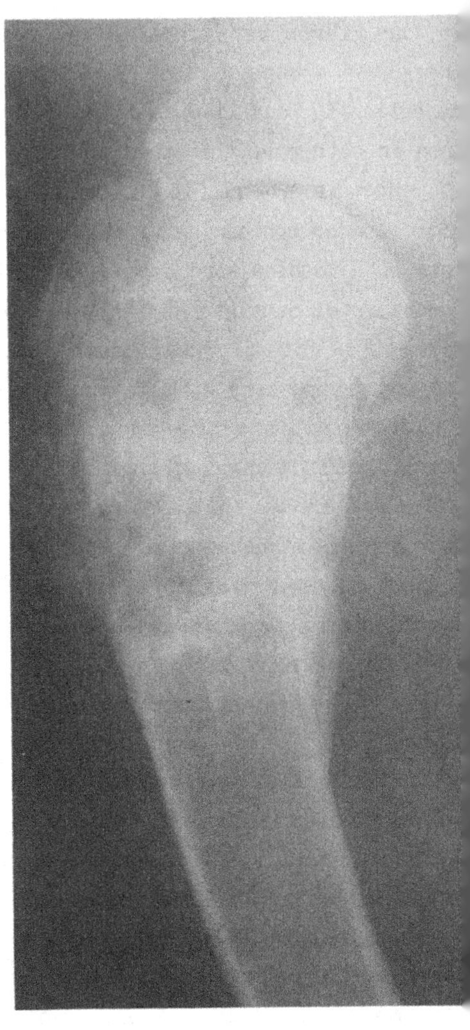

FIGURE 17

FIGURE 16. Pre-treatment radiograph of a dog with an osteogenic sarcoma of the proximal humerus.

FIGURE 17. Radiograph of the same dog shown in Figure 16, made 6 weeks after intra-arterial infusion of doxorubicin-bearing magnetic microspheres and localized with a 5-kW electromagnet placed on the craniolateral surface of the tumor. Re-ossification and remodeling of the tumor has occurred.

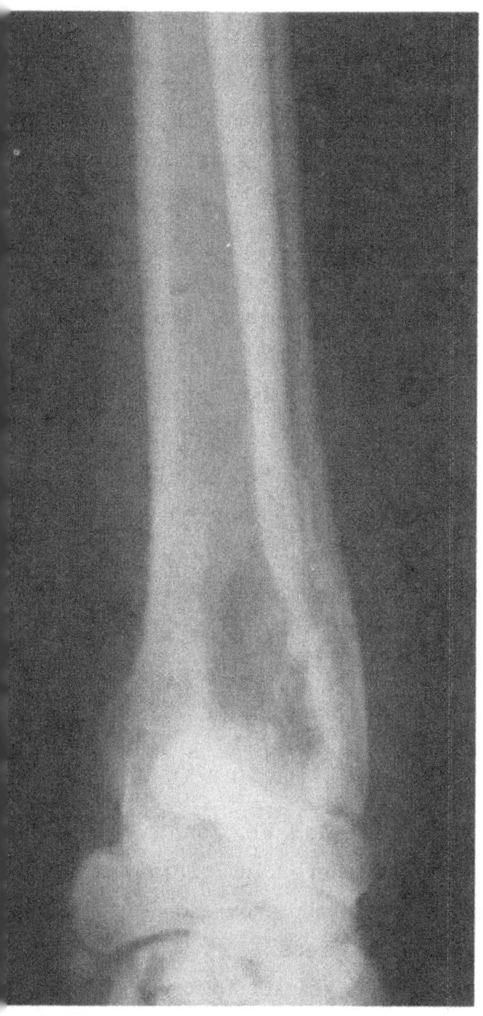

'IGURE 18

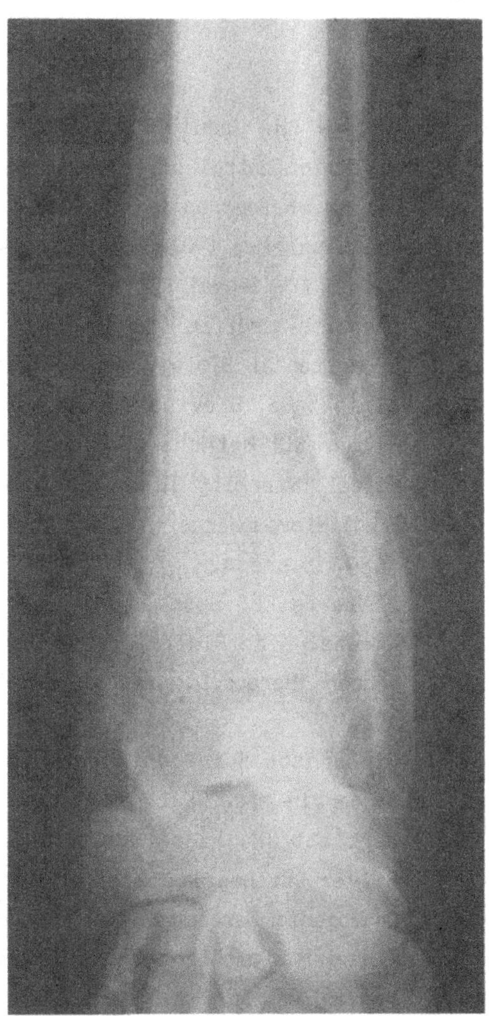

FIGURE 19

'IGURE 18. Pre-treatment radiograph of a dog with an osteogenic sarcoma of he distal radius.
'IGURE 19. Radiograph of the same dog shown in Figure 18, made 5 weeks after ntramedullary infusion of doxorubicin-bearing magnetic microspheres and ocalized with a 5-kW electromagnet placed on the dorsal aspect of the tumor. e-ossification has occurred.

Since varying experimental methods were used in this feasibility study, nd since response to therapy was not the primary problem being addressed, no onclusions regarding specific sphere/drug dosage should be drawn from our 'indings. However, 26% of the dogs treated demonstrated temporary improvement nd 15% showed measurable remission. These results provide additional hope hat magnetic drug-containing microspheres may help bring about complete emissions in patients while causing minimal damage to functions and tructures.

REFERENCES

1. Meyers PH, Cronic F, Nice CM: Experimental Approach in the Use and Magnetic Control of Metallic Iron Particles in the Lymphatic and Vascular System of Dogs as a Contrast and Isotopic Agent. Am J Roentgenol Radium Ther Nucl Med (90):1068-1077, 1963.
2. Widder KJ, Senyei AE, Scarpelli DG: Magnetic Microspheres: A Model System for Site-specific Drug Delivery in Vivo. Proceedings of the Society for Experimental Biology and Medicine, (58):141-146, 1978.
3. Elliott GS, Blevins WE, Richardson, RC, Janas W, Bartlett JM, Hale JR Silver RL: Methods of Vascular Access for Delivery of Microspheres to Distal Extremity Tumors in Dogs -- A Large-animal Model. In: Tomlinson E(ed) Microspheres and Drug Therapy. Elsevier Biomedical Press, New York 1984, in press.
4. Gillette EL: Spontaneous Canine Neoplasms as Models for Therapeutic Agents. In: Fidler IJ, White RJ (eds): Design of Models for Testing Cancer Therapeutic Agents. Van Nostrand Reinhold, New York, 1982, pp185-192.
5. Richardson RC: Spontaneous Canine and Feline Neoplasms as Models for Cancer in Man. Kal Kan Forum, (2):89-94, 1983.
6. Bartlett JM, Richardson RC, Elliott GS, Blevins WE, Janas W, Hale JR, Silver RL: Localization of Magnetic Microspheres in Thirty-six Canine Osteogenic Sarcomas. In: Tomlinson E(ed) Microspheres and Drug Therapy Elsevier Biomedical Press, New York, 1984, in press.
7. Widder KJ, Morris RM, Poore G, Howard DP, Senyei AE: Tumor Remission in Yoshida Sarcoma-bearing Rats by Selective Targeting of Magnetic Albumin Microspheres Containing Doxorubicin. Proc Natl Acad Sci USA (78):579-581, 1981.
8. Widder KJ, Morris RM, Poore GA, Howard DP, Senyei AE: Selective Targeting of Magnetic Albumin Microspheres Containing Low-dose Doxorubicin: Total Remission in Yoshida Sarcoma-bearing Rats. Eur J Cancer Clin Oncol (19):135-139, 1983.
9. Sugibayashi K, Okumura M, Morimoto Y: Biomedical Applications of Magnetic fluids III. Antitumor Effect of Magnetic Albumin Microsphere-entrapped Adriamycin on Lung Metastasis of AH 7974 in Rats. Biomaterials (3):181-186, 1982.

10. Morris RM, Poore GA, Howard DP, Sefranka JA: Selective Targeting of Magnetic Albumin Microspheres Containing Vindesine Sulfate: Total Remission in Yoshida Sarcoma-bearing Rats. In: Tomlinson E(ed) Microspheres and Drug Therapy. Elsevier Biomedical Press, New York, 1984, in press.

POLYMER IMMOBILIZED DOXORUBICIN AS A REGIONAL THERAPEUTIC AGENT

Thomas R. Tritton[1], John S. Lazo[1], Polly Lane[1], David Labaree[1], and Lemuel B. Wingard, Jr.[2]

[1] Department of Pharmacology, Yale University School of Medicine, New Haven, CT 06510 and [2] Department of Pharmacology, University of Pittsburgh School of Medicine, Pittsburgh, PA 15261.

RATIONALE

All drugs encounter cell surface membranes. Pharmacologists have been concerned with the importance of these membranes as barriers to the action of medicinal agents for many years. The enormous increase in our understanding of the composition and function of cellular membranes has, however, stimulated a variety of investigations which have shown that a number of drugs exert their pharmacological effects through direct alteration of intrinsic membrane function(s). In fact, for essentially every distinct property of cellular membranes, one can readily identify a drug which acts on that property. A few examples include fluidity (local anesthetics), overall permeability (polyene antibiotics), transport of small molecules (tricyclic antidepressants), spatial organization (antiseptic phenol), maintenance of ion gradients (digitalis), and receptor binding (benzodiazapines) (1-6). **The philosophy of the present discussion is that if a drug acts at a cell surface site, then localizing or restricting the drug to that site may increase the therapeutic specificity of the drug.** In this article we will describe a theoretical and experimental rationale for applying this concept to chemotherapy and then present some preliminary results showing a potential applicability to cancer treatment.

MECHANISMS OF ANTICANCER DRUG ACTION

There have been suggestions in the literature that certain anticancer drugs may have membranes as a primary or secondary target site. Examples include alkylating agents (7), bleomycin (8), cis-platinum (9) and actinomycin D (10). The most extensive evidence implicating a membrane site of action for an anticancer agent, however, has been with doxorubicin. The classic mechanism of action of this agent is that binding to DNA by intercalation leads to a disruption of DNA function (11). The argument supporting this hypothesis is largely structural; that is, since the drug is positively charged and contains a planar, aromatic ring system, it binds with high affinity to double-stranded DNA. Thus the action of the drug is assumed to derive from such binding. This argument is logical, since doxorubicin does accumulate in the nucleus of treated cells and since it inhibits polymerase enzymes. It has also been proposed that anthracyclines may damage DNA by alkylation or oxidative attack. These actions derive from the ability of this quinone-containing molecule to be reduced to the semiquinone, or the dihydroquinone, thereby leading to reactive alkylating species or generation of oxygen-containing radicals. The evidence for and against these various mechanisms has been discussed without resolving the issue (12,13).

There are several lines of evidence that argue against DNA as the principal target for this class of agents. First, if direct inhibition of DNA synthesis by intercalated drug was the primary reason for cytotoxic action, then one would expect to find a corresponding structure-function relationship among the hundreds of anthracycline congeners synthesized. No such relationship exists. Second, and more persuasive, is the fact that congeners have been synthesized which are cytotoxic but which have little or no affinity for DNA (e.g. AD-32 (14), carminomycin-11-methyl ether (15), N,N-dibenzyl doxorubicin (16)). Thus binding to DNA, per se, cannot be an essential requirement for the action of these drugs toward susceptible cells. Third, recent work (35, 36) has shown that there is no direct relationship between cytotoxicity and the quantitative amounts of DNA damage caused by a number of intercalators, including doxorubicin. Fourth, our laboratory has found that with doxorubicin, the effects of the drug on cell viability are not tightly coupled to inhibition of DNA or RNA synthesis (37).

Just as the structural argument was used to support a DNA target for doxorubicin, so can a structural argument be used to support a membrane target. This is because doxorubicin has the structural feature necessary for efficient interaction with cell membranes, namely, it is amphipathic. Such molecules contain both polar and non-polar character and typically possess the ability to affect both the structure and function of biological membranes. Thus, one could reasonably propose, based solely on the structure of the drug, that cell membranes could be a direct target for pharmacologic action. If this hypothesis were to be tested, two criteria could be proposed to validate the idea. First, doxorubicin would have to interact with components of membranes, and second, the drug would have demonstrable activity toward biological functions mediated by cell membranes. In fact, we (17) and others (18) have shown that doxorubicin does interact effectively with membrane phospholipids. Acidic phospholipids, particularly cardiolipin, may even provide specificity for the binding of doxorubicin when these lipids are present in a membrane bilayer (17,18).

Doxorubicin also meets the second criterion of the membrane target hypothesis: namely, it is capable of affecting numerous biological activities carried out by membranes. The first demonstration of a cell surface activity of this agent was a drug-induced increase in the agglutination rate of cells in culture by Concanavalin A (19). This initial work has led to numerous other studies showing that anthracyclines modulate plasma membrane properties. For example, we have shown that doxorubicin stimulates a rapid, dose-dependent increase in membrane fluidity as judged by spin-labeling techniques (20). Furthermore, other biological properties of the drug, such as its action on hypoxic tumor cells and its reduced action towards resistant cell lines, have also been implicated as being directly coupled to membrane fluidity (21). The morphology of membranes is also influenced by doxorubicin (22), as is the ability of membranes to act as a permeability barrier to ions such as K^+ and Ca^{2+}. In addition, such diverse membrane properties as protein glycosylation (25) and the expression of epidermal growth factor receptors (26,27) are susceptible to the influence of this anticancer drug.

POLYMER-IMMOBILIZED DOXORUBICIN

The list of membrane actions of doxorubicin and its relatives is even more extensive than indicated here (we have reviewed the area in Ref. 28), but the existence of the list does not prove that any of those membrane responses are critical for cytotoxic action. The strongest evidence that the cell surface is a primary target for doxorubicin comes from experiments using polymer-immobilized drug (29-32, 38-40). In this form doxorubicin can only interact with the cell-surface since the polymers used are larger than cells. Consequently, DNA interactions are precluded. Using doxorubicin immobilized to both agarose and polyvinyl alcohol, we have shown evidence to suggest that the drug is actively cytotoxic under conditions where it can be demonstrated that negligible free drug enters the cell. Table 1 shows some typical experimental results (29). Agarose beads without attached adriamycin are not cytotoxic and, as expected, do not reveal any intracellular drug by HPLC analysis. Native, free adriamycin causes the expected dose-dependent cell kill and the accumulated cellular content of the drug appears to correlate with cytotoxicity. A notable point here, however, is that even though 10^{-9} M adriamycin is not active, we can still detect cellular accumulation. By contrast, the polymer-immobilized adriamycin preparation is cytotoxic, but no free drug is found associated with the cells. Results obtained by a similar approach in another laboratory (38,39) are in agreement. Consequently, we conclude that an agent that was heretofore postulated to have intracellular DNA as its major target can still be active, even when restricted solely to interaction at the cell surface. Furthermore, the potential relevance for cancer treatment is emphasized by the fact that the immobilized doxorubicin appears to be 100 to 1000 times more potent than free doxorubicin, suggesting that the cell surface represents a very responsive site for drug action and that non-penetrating derivatives might be an extraordinarily useful new class of anticancer agents.

TABLE 1

Survival of L1210 clones in soft agar following exposure to free and immobilized adriamycin. The polymeric support in these experiments is agarose (~100 μm diameter) and the chemical linkage is an N-alkyl carbamate. Fifty ml of cells (1 x 10^5/ml) were exposed to the indicated treatment for two hours. The cells in one ml were assayed for cytotoxicity by cloning in soft agar and the remaining 49 ml extracted for HPLC analysis of intracellular adriamycin as previously described (29-32). The cell-associated adriamycin is given in arbitrary fluorescence units; a value of 0 means that no fluorescence could be detected.

Treatment	% Survival	Cell-Associated Adriamycin
Control cells	100	0
+ agarose	100	0
+10^{-9} M adriamycin	99	8
+5 x 10^{-8} M adriamycin	60	60
+1 x 10^{-7} M adriamycin	41	110
+50 mg agarose-adriamycin	63	0
+100 mg agarose-adriamycin	32	0

PROSPECTS FOR CLINICAL USE

It is unlikely that large polymers will prove to be of general use in the treatment of cancer because of their inability to transgress the capillary bed. Polymeric drugs may, however, be useful for neoplastic disorders in which the disease is localized in one pharmacologic compartment. Epithelial tumors of the ovary, which are the most commonly fatal gynecologic malignancy, are frequently restricted to the peritoneal region, viz FIGO Stages I-III. Likewise, ascites formation is restricted to the same anatomical area. Thus, some investigators have attempted to exploit this regional confinement by instilling drugs intraperitoneally with large volumes of fluid (33). Unfortunately, the physico-chemical properties of the currently available antitumor agents do not permit the prolonged retention of large amounts of active drug in the peritoneal cavity (34).

Cytotoxic compounds covalently linked to long polymers have a number of advantages over free drug administration (Table 2). First, the polymers have the potential of long residence times in the peritoneum and, thus, will make prolonged or sustained contact with the target cells. Second, since the drug is restricted to the exterior of cells, no intracellular degradation, sequestration or distribution will occur. Consequently, these pharmacologic variables will not complicate therapy. Third, the drug could be used at low concentrations since the *in vivo* results suggest that cell surface attack is much more potent than action at intracellular sites. The ability to use small doses might in turn obviate some of the untoward side effects of treatment using cytotoxic agents. Fourth, because the undesirable toxicities of doxorubicin (e.g. cardiac toxocity) are probably mediated at intracellular sites and at locations removed from the peritoneum, such side effects could be avoided with the non-penetrating drug-polymer complex.

TABLE 2

ADVANTAGES OF INTRAPERITONEAL ADMINISTRATION OF IMMOBILIZED DRUGS
Prolonged contact with target
Little metabolism or degradation
Low concentration
No intracellular toxicity

The considerations presented so far suggest that a persuasive rationale exists for the design of non-penetrating cytotoxic agents for the treatment of cancer. We are particularly interested in the use of solid-phase immobilized doxorubicin as a potential modality for intracavitary therapy of ovarian epithelial malignancies, or to treat ascites forms of cancer. Animal model systems exist for these cases; some prelimiary experimental results obtained with the mouse ascites, L1210 model are summarized in Table 3. This tumor is only moderately sensitive to free adriamycin when the drug is given as a single i.p. injection. Immobilized adriamycin at the same total dose causes about the same increase in survival as free drug. However, the effective dose of the immobilized drug is much lower than the total dose since most of the drug is inside the polymer and thus presumably unavailable to cellular contact. It is possible that the polymeric form simply acts as a sustained depot for free adriamycin. We think this is unlikely, however, for two reasons. First, a slow release of a low level of drug would probably not be effective as an antitumor agent. Second, the polymer-treated animals do not suffer any weight loss when compared to untreated animals. In contrast, animals treated with the same total dose of free adriamycin experience significant weight loss (~40% as compared to controls) due to the presence of the cytotoxic agent. Thus, the antitumor effect of the immobilized drug appears to be due to direct action of the polymer-bound species.

TABLE 3
EFFECTS OF SINGLE I.P. DOSE vs. L1210 CELLS IN C57Bl/6N MICE

	free adriamycin	immobilized adriamycin
survial, % increase	20-50% 2.5-13 mg/kg	33 % 4 mg/kg total
toxicity	numerous	minimal
weight loss compared to controls	yes	no

One hundred thousand viable tumor cells were implanted intraperitoneally on day one, along with either free or immobilized adriamycin or underivatized polymer. The injection volume was 1-2 ml; the polymer dose was up to 200 mg per animal to match the total doxorubicin to a 4 mg/kg dose if given as a free drug. No acute toxicity has been observed either to the large injection volume or to the presence of agarose or polyvinyl alcohol polymers in the peritoneal region. After 60 davs a 20%

increase in the weight of the spleens of treated animals has been observed. The significance of this is not yet known. The animals were given food and water *ad lib.* and weighed daily until death (11.4 ± 1.1 days for untreated tumor-bearing animals). Antitumor activity is calculated as the mean percent increase in survival, compared to untreated controls.

We have been unable to detect any acute toxic repercussions of intraperitoneal polymer administration of agarose beads containing or lacking bound doxorubicin. No focal damage or gross adhesions on the peritoneal wall of mice exposed to doxorubicin beads for periods of up to 60 days have been observed. Histological analyses of peritoneal organs and hearts of treated mice are currently being evaluated. Thus, our preliminary results strongly support the idea that cell surface-directed regional chemotherapy using immobilized drugs can be both effective and less toxic when compared to native drug.

References

1. Pang, K.Y., Chang, T.-L., and Miller, D.W. *Mol. Pharm.* *15*, 729 (1980).
2. Archer, D.B. *Biochem. Biophys. Res. Comm.* *66*, 195 (1975).
3. Talvenheimo, J., Nelson, P.J. and Rudnick, G. *J. Biol. Chem.* *254*, 4631 (1979).
4. Lambert, P.A. *Prog. Med. Chem.* *15*, 88 (1978).
5. Ahera, T., Larsen, F.S. and Brady, T.M. *J. Pharm. Exp. Therap.* *173*, 145 (1970).
6. Squires, R.F. and Braestrup, C. *Nature* *266*, 732 (1977).
7. Ihlenfeldt, M., Gantner, G., Harrer, M., Puschendeif, B., Putzer, H. and Grunicke, H. *Cancer Res.* *41*, 289 (1981).
8. Mizuno, S. and Ishida, A. *Cancer Res.* *42*, 4726 (1982).
9. Scanlon, K., Safirstein, R.L., Thies, M., Gross, R.B., Waxman, S. and Gutan, J.B., *Cancer Res.* *43*, 4211 (1983).
10. Fico, R.M., Chen, T.-K. and Canellakis, E.S. *Science* *198*, 53 (1977).
11. DiMarco, A., Soldati, A., Fioretti, A. and Dasdia, T. *Tumori* *49*, 235 (1963).
12. Favaudon, V. *Biochimie* *64*, 457 (1982).
13. Kennedy, K.A., Siegfried, J.M., Sartorelli, A.C. and Tritton, T.R. *Cancer Res.* *43*, 54 (1983).
14. Sengupta, S.K., Shehadri, R., Modest, E.J. and Israel, M. *Proc. Amer. Assoc. Cancer Res.* *17*, 109 (1976).
15. DuVernay, V.H. and Crooke, S.T. in *Anthracyclines: Current Status and New Developments*, Crooke, S.T. and Reich, S.D., eds. Academic Press, N.Y., p. 61 (1980).
16. Acton, E.M. *op cit.*, p. 11 (1980).
17. Tritton, T.R., Murphree, S.A. and Sartorelli, A.C. *Biochem.*

Biophys. Res. Comm. 84, 802 (1978).
18. Duarte-Karim, M., Ruysschaert, J.M. and Hildebrand, J. Biochem. Biophys. Res. Comm. 71, 658 (1976)
19. Murphree, S.A., Cunningham, L.S., Hwang, K.M. and Sartorelli, A.C. Biochem. Pharm. 26, 2319 (1976).
20. Murphree, S.A., Tritton, T.R., Smith, P.L. and Sartorelli, A.C. Biochim. Biophys. Acta 649, 317 (1981).
21. Siegfried, J.A., Kennedy, K.A., Sartorelli, A.C. and Tritton, T.R. J. Biol. Chem. 258, 339 (1983).
22. Mikkelson, R.B., Lin, P.-S. and Wallach, D.F.H. J. Mol. Med. 2, 33 (1977).
23. Harper, J.R., Orringer, E.P. and Parker, J.C. Res. Comm. Chem. Path. Pharm. 26, 277 (1979).
24. Dasdia, T., DiMarco, A., Goffredi, M., Minghetti, A. and Necco, A. Pharm. Res. Comm. 11, 19 (1979).
25. Kessel, D. Mol. Pharm. 16, 306 (1979).
26. Zuckier, G., Tomiko, S. and Tritton, T.R. Fed. Proc. 40, 1877 (1981).
27. Zuckier, G. and Tritton, T.R., Exp. Cell Res. 148, 155 (1983).
28. Tritton, T.R. and Hickman, J.A. in Oncology series: Chemotherapy Vol. II, William L. McGuire, Ed., in press (1983).
29. Tritton, T.R. and Yee, G. Science 217, 248 (1982).
30. Tritton, T.R., Wingard, L. and Yee, G., symposium in Fed. Proc. 42, 284 (1983).
31. Wingard, L. and Tritton, T.R., in Affinity Chromatography and Biological Recognition, Chaiken, J.M., Wilcheck, M. and Parikh, I. (eds.) Academic Press (1983).
32. Wingard, L. and Tritton, T.R., Manuscript in preparation.
33. Ozols, R.F., Young, R.C., Speyer, J.L., Sugarbaker, P.h., Greene, R., Jenkins, J. and Myers, C.E. Cancer Res. 42, 4265 (1982).
34. Jones, R.B., Myers, C.E., Guarino, A.M., Dedrick, R.L., Hubbard, S.M., and DeVita, V.T., Cancer Chemother. Pharm. 1, 161 (1970).
35. Zwelling, L.A., Kerrigan, D. and Michaels, S. Cancer Res. 42, 2687 (1982).
36. Pommier, Y., Zwelling, L.A., Mattern, M.R., Erickson, L.C., Kerrigan, D., Schwartz, R. and Kohn, K.W. Cancer Res. 43, 5718 (1983).
37. Siegfried, J., Sartorelli, A.C. and Tritton, T.R. Cancer Biochem. Biophys. 6, 137 (1983).
38. Tokes, Z.A., Rogers, K.E. and Rembaum, A. Proc. Nat. Acad. Sci. 79, 2026 (1982).
39. Rogers, K.E., Carr, B.J., and Tokes, Z.A. Cancer Res. 43, 2741 (1983).
40. Wingard, L.B. Biochem. Pharm. 32, 2647 (1983).

Acknowledgements: We thank the NIH (CA 28852 and RR 05416) and American Cancer Society (CH-212, CH-174 and IN-58S) for financial support. TRT is the recipient of a Research Career Development Award (CA 00684).

THE USE OF RADIOLABELED ANTIBODY IN CANCER CHEMOTHERAPY

S.E. ORDER

INTRODUCTION

Unavailable in the radiation armamentarium of modern day oncology are systemic and highly specific agents for selective radiation. Radiolabeled antibodies now offer both the specific selectivity as well as the opportunity for selective systemic irradiation which may be enhanced by appropriate chemotherapeutic integration.

In this newly developing modality,radiolabeled antibodies important observations have begun to be defined that are necessary to understand both for the restrictions and the promise they hold for future applications.

THE PHYSICS OF RADIOLABELED ANTIBODY

Our laboratory has demonstrated with I-131 antiferritin that dose escalation is inappropriate in the treatment of hepatoma and that "tumor saturation" may be achieved with as little as 30mCi of I-131 antiferritin (1). Higher doses of the radiolabeled antibody would only mean greater systemic,rather than selective, radiation. The toxicity of the I-131 antiferritin is thrombocytopenia (2), and higher doses of radiation would mean greater hematologic suppression. It will therefore be necessary in the use of other antibody specificities to avoid excessive dose and to establish the dose for tumor saturation (Table 1).

TABLE 1. PHYSICS OF RADIOLABELLED ANTIBODY

	Goal	Result
Dose Administered	Tumor Saturation	Restrictive Toxicity
Type of Antibody Preparation (species; molecular state)	Tumor Effective Half life	Maximize Tumor Radiation Dose
Isotope Label	Restrictive but Effective Cytotoxicity	Selective Tumor Cell Destruction

During our investigation of various species of animals as sources for the I-131 antiferritin antibody, the demonstration that tumor effective half-life (a product of the biologic and physical half-life of the radiolabeled antibody) varied with species of origin became apparent. These findings relate to the biological degradation of the various immunoglobulins. To date, rabbit, pig, and monkey antibodies are superior to goat, chicken sheep, turkey, and bovine species. Why should this be of importance? The radiation dose is determined by the tumor effective half-life (Table 1).

In our experience to date, affinity chromatography-purified antibody (3) and antibody fragments both have reduced tumor effective half-lives. It is particularly important to realize that Fab or Fab^2 may be excellent for diagnostic purposes becaus of rapid clearance of nonspecific antibody and therefore a bette background to foreground ratio; however this does not imply that these fragments are as effective for therapeutic purposes. Fab and Fab^2 are not effective due to the abbreviated tumor effective half-lives and lessened tumor dose (4).

In discussing the selection of a radiolabel, I-131 was an excellent isotope for initial studies due to the traditional experience of the use of this isotope in thyroid cancer. The gamma component of I-131 allows visualization by scanning, and the beta component carries out the cytotoxic treatment (5). However monoclonal antibodies of high specific activity when labeled with I-131 are readily dehalogenated (6). Dehalogenation of I-131 labeled monoclonal antibodies reduces their potential as active agents for therapy. In addition, outpatient therapy, a long term goal, cannot be achieved in a significant number of malignancies. A variety of beta-emitting isotopes now being studied would allow monoclonal and polyclonal outpatient treatment. These isotopes, depending on their energy, would yield new dose rates and alter the kinetics of radiolabeled antibody administration.

If the hepatoma experience is used as a model, the tumor saturation is 30mCi, and the tumor effective half life 4-5 days. Two infusions--day 0, 30mCi,and day 5, 20mCi-- yield 1000-1200 rad of continuous irradiation. These latter observations allow one to introduce the radiobiology of radiolabeled antibody as the next step toward integration of radiolabeled antibodies in oncologic practice.

RADIOBIOLOGY OF RADIOLABELED ANTIBODIES

An important difference between radiolabeled antibody irradiation and conventional external irradiation is the continuous nature of low dose rates with radiolabeled antibody. Shipley (7) demonstrated that low dose rate irradiation at 10, 15, and 30 rad/hour,if administered to the same total dose, led to similar cell destruction in a Lewis lung carcinoma. However, the tumor mass was larger at the lower dose rates due to cellular proliferation occurring in the more prolonged time needed to achieve equivalent total tumor doses at the lower dose rates. Tumor cell destruction was continuous with continuous low dose rate irradiation. The best clinical example is the use of I-125 seeds in prostate cancer, which achieved 5-15 rad/hour (8). In the application of radiolabeled antibody in hepatoma, 5-7 rad per hour was achieved (Table 2).

TABLE 2. RADIOBIOLOGY OF RADIOLABELED ANTIBODY

	Goal	Result
Isotope Energy + Tumor Effective Half-life	Tumor Dose Rate Total Tumor Dose	Tumor Regression
Antibody	Immunologic Radiosensitization Macrophage Activation	Tumor Regression Enhanced
Adriamycin + 5 Fluorouracil	Enhanced-Dose Cytotoxicity	Increased Regression

The radiobiology of isotope -labeled antibody is not restricted to dose rate effects, since macrophage activation was shown to be cytotoxic in the experimental treatment of ovarian cancer with antibody(9,10). During the treatment of some hepatoma patients, recycling of a radiolabeled antibody previously used for treatment has led, in some patients, to rapi immmunologic clearance and reduction of tumor effective half-lives from 3-4 days to 1 day or less. This clearly indicates that sensitization had occurred during the first cycle of the same preparation. Considering that a day 0 and a day 5 infusion were carried out with a tumor effective half-life of 4-5 days, and that one month of exposure to the foreign protein occured, this was not surprising.

Suit has reported that immunogenic tumors also have a reduce Tcd50 (tumor control dose for 50% of the animals) compared to non-immunogenic tumors (11). On several occasions during his sabbatical, Dr. Baral of the Karolinska Institute measured some increased NK cell activity in our radiolabeled antibody-treated patients following administration of radiolabeled antibody (Tabl 2).

Adriamycin and 5FU have been reported to be cytoactive drugs in the treatment of hepatoma (12). Adriamycin was shown to increase the cytotoxic effects of low dose rate radiation (13), and 5FU was shown in clinical studies to amplify therapeutic effectiveness when combined with irradiation (14). In our hepatoma studies, the combination of I-131 antiferritin + 15mg of Adriamycin and 500mg 5FU has been documented to lead to a 50% partial remission rate. Remission has been evaluated not by physical examination alone but rather by tumor volume reconstruction. How is tumor volume reconstruction carried out? Serial C.T. scans taken 1cm apart are reconstructed after analysis by a diagnostic radiologist and then placed in a second computer which determines the volume of tumor and total liver volume (FIGURE 1.). Partial remission is defined as a 30% or greater reduction in volume. Fifty percent of hepatoma patients have remitted during the phase 1-2 trial.

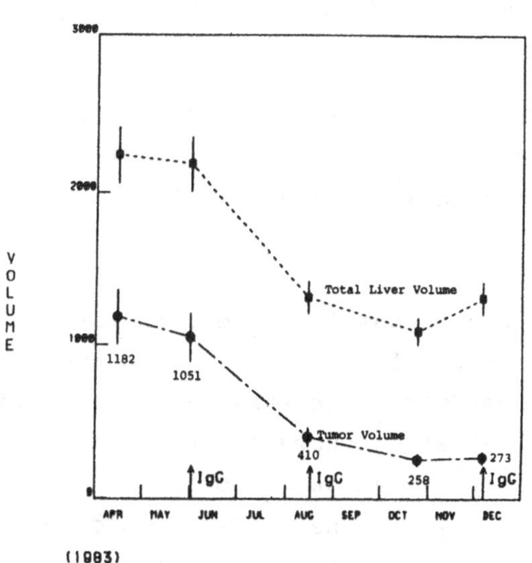

FIGURE 1.a) Total liver volume and tumor volume (dashed line) plotted by reconstruction of 1cm CT scans throughout the entire liver.

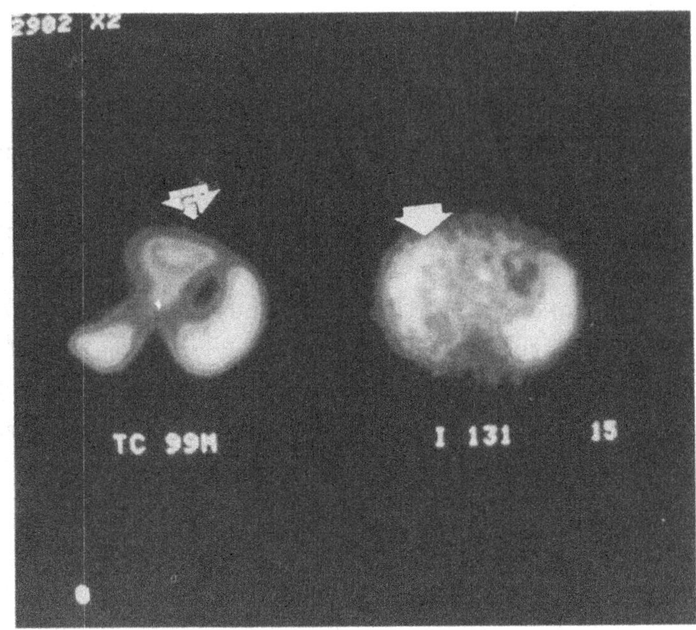

FIGURE 1.b) Tc^{99m} sulfur colloid tomographic nuclear scan demonstrates minimal uptake in spleen. The I-131 antiferritin tomographic nuclear scan is at the same level and shows tumor uptake.

Shipley (7) in his continuous low-dose irradiation experiments demonstrated that tumor cell cytotoxicity is equivalent at equivalent total tumor doses but takes a longer period of time t achieve at lower dose rates. However, he further demonstrated that if tumor cell proliferation were occurring during this prolonged period of time the net effect would be tumor expansion. In our phase 1-2 study, we noted that patients with AFP + hepatomas seemed to have more virulent and rapidly expanding tumors. Of 100 patients who received at least 1 cycle of radiolabeled antibody, the median survival of AFP + (47 patients) was 6 months, and AFP- (53 patients) 11 months. This i consistent with the concept that cell proliferation is not rapid and that the net effect of low dose rate radiation leads to tumo regression.

CHARACTERISTICS OF TUMOR TARGETING BY RADIOLABELED ANTIBODY

This is a complex problem. If an antigen is present in a cancer, and if radiolabeled antibody deposits in the tumor, it is not necessarily a potential therapeutic agent. For example, alpha fetoprotein, although present in hepatoma when used as a target for I-131 antiAFP, reveals tumor adherence,but the concentration of antiAFP persisting at the tumor target is not sufficient for therapeutic purposes (Table 3).

TABLE 3. RADIOIMMUNOGLOBULIN TUMOR DEPOSITION

Hepatoma	^{131}I AFP 2.7μCi/gm ^{131}I Antiferritin 7.3μCi/gm
Intrahepatic Biliary Cancer	^{131}I AntiCEA 4.7μCi/gm

Similarly, a trial with I-131 antiCEA demonstrated a 40-50% response rate in intrahepatic biliary cancer and no significant response in colorectal cancer metastatic to the liver. Therefore, assumptions often made that a tumor-normal-tissue ratio represents "tumor targeting" of potential therapeutic value is incorrect. These "ratios" often used in Nuclear Medicine are meaningful in regard to the ability to scan and may be achieved by using Fab or Fab^2 fragments which wash out of background rapidly, thereby leaving foreground tumor more visible. However, increased tumor concentration of therapeutic significance (μCi/gm) over time (tumor effective half-life) is not an automatic product of the scanning assumption. The confusing relationship of increased apparent tumor signal due to decreased background does not mean increased tumor dose deposition over time (15). Further, a 1% or less deposition of radiolabeled antibody activity in tumor,although yielding positive tumor scanning, again would be limited as to therapeutic value due to nonbound circulating radiolabeled antibody(16). Our investigative team has therefore developed criteria for radiolabeled antibody for therapeutic purposes (Table 4).

TABLE 4. CRITERIA FOR RADIOLABELLED ANTIBODY FOR THERAPEUTIC PURPOSES

Tumor Selectivity "in vivo"
Concentration at Tumor in µCi/gm
Tumor Effective Half-life
Tumor Dose (rad)
Remission/Toxicity Ratio

Even within a tumor class bearing an antigen known to bind a radiolabeled antibody, for example I-131 Antiferritin in hepatoma there are new principles of therapeutic targeting. Dr. Robert Rostock demonstrated in an H42e hepatoma that ferritin synthesis decreases with increasing tumor size and that tumor vascularity decreases with increasing tumor size (17, 18). Therefore, the efficiency of tumor targeting is maximized with small tumors wit increased ferritin synthesis and abundant neovasculature. These characteristics seem to allow for the preferential binding of I-131 Antiferritin and have been designated the "biologic window". The supposition that radiolabeled antibody must target unique, or so called "tumor specific" antigens is not a necessar requirement. The tumor deposition with I-131 AntiCEA also represents binding of a tumor-associated antigen where the antigenic moiety emanates from the cells into the stroma and circulation, causing a measurable titer to be apparent. Whether the relationships for the "biologic window" are similar or dissimilar for other antigenic moieties remains to be studied.

Finally, in those antigens restricted to tumor tissue and normal tissue but not circulating, the opportunities for tumor dose deposition most likely will have other variables influencin the successful application of these radiolabeled antibodies.

MULTIPLE TARGET ANTIGENS

During the early development of radiolabeled antibody for cancer therapy, we have begun to explore in nonresectable lung cancers which have ferritin and CEA the dual targeting of both antigenic moieties simultaneously. Although it is too early in development to warrant conclusion as to dose amplification, successful dual targeting has been achieved (FIGURE 2).

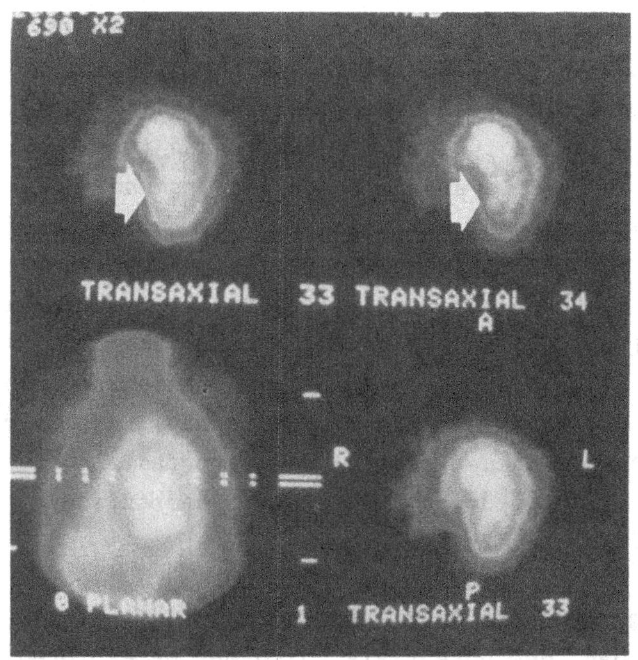

FIGURE 2. An anterior-posterior nuclear scan converted by circumferential nuclear scanning and computer-directed tomographic reconstruction into transaxial views and demonstrating localization of I-131 anti-CEA and antiferritin in a left upper lobe lesion.

The importance of dual-targeting is the potential increase in the concentration of radiolabeled antibody deposited in the tumor and the opportunity to amplify tumor dose and, therefore, tumor cytotoxicity.

CLINICAL APPLICATION OF RADIOLABELED ANTIBODY

Our composite experience in over 200 patients has demonstrated with polyclonal antibodies no acute toxicity but thrombocytopenia which is both dose dependent and dependent on integration with chemotherapy. Cyclic treatment by altering species of antibody derivation has been feasible (19). Monoclonal antibody radiolabeled with I-131 has been dehalogenated in vivo. Depending on the dose of I-131, radiolabeled antibody has been administered to both inpatients and outpatients and is easily accomplished in the clinic. Early results of our trials are in Hodgkin's disease (MOPP + ABVD failures): 40% partial remission and 73% remission of B symptoms (20): hepatoma and intrahepatic biliary cancer,40-50% partial remission have been reported (21,22). All results have been multi-institutional and sponsored through the RTOG (Radiation Therapy Oncology Group). Presently, a randomized prospective trial in hepatoma is comparing chemotherapy, Adriamycin, 60mg/M^2 and 5FU, 500mg/M^2 given every 3 weeks to radiolabeled I-131 Antiferritin, 30mCi day 0, 20mCi day 5 and Adriamycin, 15mg and 5FU, 500mg given every 2 months.

FUTURE DIRECTIONS AND DEVELOPMENTS

Of the many new potentials which may be explored, two remain the most immediate needs.

The automation of dosimetry for radiolabeled antibody in a conjoint program with Hirsch-Chemie will allow rapid development of:

1. Proper prescription of radiolabeled antibody dose.
2. Evaluation of simultaneous, multiple-specificity radiolabeled antibodies in therapy.
3. Selection of best radiolabeled antibodies (mono-

clonal and polyclonal).

4. Evaluation of radioimmunotherapeutic treatment.

The development of a new therapeutic radiolabel effective for both monoclonal and polyclonal antibodies--in a conjoint effort with Hybritech, Inc.--will allow:

1. Predominantly outpatient treatment (beta emission with minimal gamma signal).
2. Escalation of dose rate and possibly total tumor dose for increased therapeutic effectiveness.
3. Intercomparisons of dosimetry of multiple monoclonal and polyclonal antibodies.

The development of new specificities is today far less challenging since the advent of hybridoma monoclonal technology, which allows identification and restriction of antigenic moieties at a rapid pace (23).

The integration of radiolabeled antibodies with chemotherapy should significantly increase therapeutic effectiveness once dosimetry and the best radiolabeled antibody preparations are established.

In summary, our experience based on standard laboratory and clinical evaluation indicates that radiolabeled antibody has arrived as a new clinical entity, one that requires further development to fulfill its ultimate promise and place in the clinical practice of oncology.

REFERENCES:

1. Leichner, P. K., Klein, J. L., Garrison, J. B., Jenkins, R. E., Nickloff, E. L., Ettinger, D. S., Order, S. E.: Dosimetr of I-131 labeled antiferritin in hepatoma: A model for radio immunoglobulin dosimetry. Int J Rad Onc Biol Phy (7): 323-333, 1981.
2. Ettinger, D. S., Order, S. E., Wharam, M. D., Parker, M. Klein, J. L., Leichner, P. K.: Phase I-II study of isotopic immunoglobulin therapy for primary liver cancer. Cancer Trea Rep. (66): 289-297, 1982.
3. Order, S. E.: Monoclonal antibodies: Potential role in radiation therapy and oncology. Int J Rad Onc Biol Phys (8): 1193-1201, 1982.
4. Wright, T., Sinanan, M., Harrington, D., Klein, J. L., Order S.E.: Immunoglobulin: Applications to scanning and treatment Applied Rad (8) 120-124, 1979.
5. Maxon, H. R., Thomas, S. R., Hertzberg, V. S., Kereiakes, J G., Chen, I. W. Sperling, M. I., Saenger, E. L.: Relation between effective radiation dose and outcome of radioiodine therapy for thyroid cancer. New Eng J Med (309) 937-941, 1983.
6. Order, S. E.: Radioimmunoglobulin therapy of cancer. Comprehensive Therapy (10): 9-18, 1984.
7. Shipley, W. U., Peacock, J. H., Steel, G. G., Stephens, T. C.: Continuous irradiation of the Lewis lung carcinoma in vivo at clinically used "ultra" low dose rates. Int J Rad On Biol Phys (9) 1647-1653, 1983.
8. Hilaris, B.S., Whitmore, W.F., Batata, M., Barzell, W.: Behavorial patterns of prostate adenocarcinoma following an I-125 implant and pelvic lymphadenectomy. Int J Rad Onc Biol Phys (2) 631-637, 1977.
9. Feldman, G. B., Knapp, R. C., Order, S. E., Hellman, S.: The Role of lymphatic obstruction in the formation of ascites in a murine ovarian carcinoma. Cancer Res (32) 1663-1666, 1972
10. Order, S. E., Donahue, V., Knapp, R.: Immunotherapy of ovarian carcinoma. An experimental model. Cancer (32) 573-579, 1973.
11. Suit, H., Order, S.E.: Considerations in the interactions of radiation and immunotherapy. In interaction of radiation and host immune defense mechanisms in malignancy. Brookhaven National Laboratory. New York, 1974, pp. 130-151.
12. Baker, L. H., Saiki, J. A., Jones, S.A.: Adriamycin and 5-fluorouracil in the treatment of advanced hepatoma: A SW onc group study. Cancer Treat Rep (61): 1595-1598, 1977.
13. Sherman, D. M., Carabell, S.C., Belli, J. A., Hellman S.: Th effect of dose rate and adriamycin on the tolerance of thoracic radiation in mice. Int J Rad Onc Biol Phys (8): 45-51, 1982.
14. Moertel, C. G., Childs, Jr., D. S., Reitemeier, R. J., Colby Jr., M. Y., Holbrook, M. A.: Combined 5-fluorouracil and supervoltage radiation therapy of locally unresectable gastrointestinal cancer. The Lancet: 865-867, 1969.

15. Mach, J. P., Chatal, J.F., Lumbroso, S.D., Bacheggi, F., Forni, M., Pitchard, J., Beiche, C., Douillard, J. Y., Carrel, S., Herlyn, M., Steplewski, Z, Koprowski, H.: Tumor localization in patients by radiolabelled monoclonal antibodies against colon carcinoma. Cancer Res (43) 5593-5600, 1983.
16. Epenetos, A. A., Britton, K. E., Mather, S., Sheperd, J., Granowska, M., Taylor-Papadimitriou, J., Nimmon C. C., Durbin, H., Hawkins, L. R., Malpas. J. S., Bodmer, W. F.: Targeting of iodine-123 labelled tumor-associated monoclonal antibodies to ovarian, breast, and gastrointestinal tumors. Lancet (6) 999-1005, 1982.
17. Rostock, R. A., Klein, J. L., Leichner, P. K., Kopher, K. A., Order, S.E.: Selective tumor localization in experimental hepatoma by radiolabeled antiferritin antibody. Int J Rad Onc Biol Phys (9) 1345-1350, 1983.
18. Rostock, R. A., Klein, J. L., Kopher, K. A., Order, S.E.: Variables affecting the tumor localization of I-131 antiferritin in experimental hepatoma. Amer J Cl Onc (in press).
19. Order, S. E., Ettinger, D. S., Leibel, S. A., Klein, J. L., Leichner, P. K.: Cyclic radiolabeled I-131 antiferritin in multimodality therapy of hepatocellular carcinoma. Proc Amer Soc Cl Onc (2) 119, 1983.
20. Lenhard, R. E., Order, S. E., Spunberg, J. J., Ettinger, D. S., Asbell, S. O., Leibel, S. A.: Radioimmunoglobulins: A new therapeutic modality in Hodgkin s disease. Proc Amer Soc Cl Onc (2) 211, 1983.
21. Order, S. E., Klein, J. L., Ettinger, D., Alderson, P., Siegelman, S., Leichner, P.: Phase I-II study of radiolabeled antibody integrated in the treatment of primary hepatic malignancies. Int J Rad Onc Biol Phys (6): 703-710, 1980.
22. Order, S. E., Klein, J. L., Leichner, P. K., Wharam, M.D., Chambers, J., Kopher, K., Ettinger, D. S., Siegelman, S.S.: Radiolabeled antibodies in the treatment of primary liver malignancies. In: Levin, B. Riddel, R. (eds) Gastrointestinal Cancer. Elsevier North-Holland, New York (in press).
23. Kohler, G., Howe, S. C., Milstein, C.: Fusion between immunoglobulin-nonsecreting myeloma cell lines. Eur J Immunol (6) 292-295, 1976.

ACKNOWLEDGEMENTS

AMERICAN CANCER SOCIETY - PDT 227

NATIONAL CANCER INSTITUTE, RADIATION THERAPY ONCOLOGY GROUP - CA 295-36-03

NATIONAL CANCER INSTITUTE, REGIONAL ONCOLOGY CENTER SUPPORT GRANT - CA 069-73-21

INTRACAVITARY HYPERTHERMIA AND INTRA-ARTERIAL CHEMOTHERAPY

STEPHEN C. JACOBS, M.D.

Intra-arterial (IA) chemotherapy improves the therapeutic index of administered agents. This conference has addressed this issue in great depth, and I would like to comment only on the agents doxorubicin (ADR) and cis-diamminedichloroplatinum II (CDDP). ADR has been found to be more effective in the rabbit VX-2 tumor when given IA than IV.[1] ADR IA infusion of the dog limb results in greater normal tissue uptake of ADR than IV infusion.[2] Clinical IA infusions of ADR alone have shown promise for a number of tumors.[3,4] The long plasma half-life of ADR, however, would favor the IV use of this agent.[5]

CDDP has a short free half-life in plasma, and IA administration results in increased regional exposure in the infused area.[6]

Table 1: Clinical Experiences with Intra-Arterial Cisplatin

Tumor	CDDP dose	Infusion time	Author
Cervix	120 mg/m^2	2 hrs	Carlson[7]
Liver	100-120 mg/m^2	.8-23 hrs	Stewart[6]
Liver	120 mg/m^2	2 hrs	Cheng[8]
Head & Neck	50 mg/m^2	bolus	Baker[*9]
Head & Neck		2 hrs	Horiuchi[10]
Skin	90 mg/m^2	2 hrs	Ajani[11]
Osteosarcoma	100-150 mg/m^2	2 hrs	Jaffe[12]
Osteosarcoma	75-150 mg/m^2	3-4 hrs	Calvo[13]
Brain	60-120 mg/m^2	.8-1.3 hrs	Stewart[14]
Sarcoma	90-120 mg/m^2	1.5-3 hrs	Calvo[13], Stewart[6]
Breast	75-150 mg/m^2	3-4 hrs	Calvo[13]
Pelvic Cancer	60-120 mg/m^2	2.3-26 hrs	Stewart[6]
Melanoma	75-150 mg/m^2	3-4 hrs	Calvo[13], Pritchard[15]
Bladder	80-120 mg/m^2	24 hrs	Wallace[16]

*in combination with IA 5FU

The hypogastric arteries provide the major arterial supply for the deep pelvis. The take-off from the common iliac artery on each side is usually easily accessible via a percutaneous femoral approach from the contralateral side. The posterior trunk of the hypogastric artery supplies the buttocks via the superior gluteal artery. Placement of the arterial catheter beyond this vessel will increase the efficiency of IA infusion. There is a great deal of cross-perfusion in the pelvis, so that bilateral hypogastric artery catheterization is recommended. Attempts have been made to provide isolated pelvic perfusion, but the venous anastomoses in the pelvis are extensive. Spillover into the systemic circulation will certainly occur in pelvic perfusions.

Hyperthermia alone kills tumor cells by a complex mechanism involving both cell membrane permeability changes and nucleic acid and protein damage. Dewey et al[17] proposed that during hyperthermia rapidly dividing cells accummulate nuclear proteins around single-stranded regions of DNA, preventing normal DNA synthesis. Gerner[18] has proposed a second model for hyperthermic cell death that has heat causing an interaction between the polyamines and membrane cholesterol or transmembrane proteins to produce an inappropriately permeable cell membrane. In vivo, actual tumor cell killing occurs above 41.5C and increases geometrically with each degree C up to 45C. Normal cells are more resistant to hyperthermia by at least a factor of 2.

At the tissue level, tumors are unable to dissipate heat as well as normal tissues. Normal tissues respond to thermal injury by vasodilation and increasing vascular permeability, with a resultant increase in blood volume and blood flow both during and after hyperthermia. Tumor vasculature is already fully dilated and cannot augment blood flow when exposed to hyperthermia and, therefore, tumors heat more rapidly and to higher temperatures. Low tissue oxygen levels, poor nutritional conditions, and acidic pH within tumors may accelerate damage to the tumor vasculature that occurs with hyperthermia[19].

Hyperthermia and chemotherapeutic agents are synergistic in killing tumor cells both in vivo and in vitro. ADR is able to enter cells in culture more readily at elevated temperatures. Further, low tumor temperatures make cells resistant to ADR.[20,21] Permeability may be the determining factor in the effectivness of ADR. Hahn[22] and Marmor[23] have shown that in vivo killing of mouse EMT 6 sarcomas by ADR is enhanced by hyperthermia, but only at high ADR dosage. Hahn[24] went on to show that the ADR/hyperthermia relationship was quite complex. As the duration of hyperthermia increased, cells became highly resistant to ADR. The mechanisms underlying this thermally induced drug tolerance are not known.

In vitro, hyperthermia potentiates CDDP binding to cellular DNA and increases DNA cross-linking.[25,26,27] Cell killing by CDDP also increases with increasing temperature. Alberts et al.[28] showed that in an in vivo mouse model hyperthermia potentiated the anti-leukemic effect of CDDP but not its toxicity to normal marrow. Uptake of CDDP was enhanced only by hyperthermia applied just before or during exposure to CDDP. Each degree of temperature rise resulted in one log increase in tumor cell killing, suggesting that the highest possible temperatures would be most effective.

Local hyperthermia can produce higher temperatures more safely than systemic hyperthermia. Methods for applying local hyperthermia include radiowaves, microwaves, ultrasound, water baths, and heated perfusions. Each of these methods has advantages and disadvantages. Perfusion of heated blood is effective in producing hyperthermia if both the arterial inflow and venous outflow can be isolated. Limbs can be isolation-perfused quite effectively.

Table 2: Hyperthermia/isolation-perfusion trials.

Tumor	Drug	Temperature	Time	Author
Abdomen	Cytoxan Melphalan Nitrogen mustard	41-42C	1/3-1/2 hr	Shingelton[37]
Liver		42C	4 hrs	Quebbman[29]
Limb Melanoma	Melphalan	42C	1/2-2 hrs	Cavaliere [30]
Limb Osteosarcoma	Melphalan Actinomycin D	42C	1/2-2 hrs	Cavaliere [30]
Pelvis	5FU	42C	3/4 hrs	Wile[35]
Limb	CDDP	40C	1-1 1/4 hrs	Hild[31]
Melanoma	Melphalan	38.5-43C	1-1 1/4 hrs	Multiple Reviewed by Rege[34]

Surface heating can be applied for longer periods of time. Heating of the bladder from the interior is attractive because of its easy accessibility. Hall et al.[32] first applied local bladder hyperthermia by pump circulation of heated fluid to the bladder in the early 1970's. He found that 45C on the bladder luminal surface was moderately effective in destroying superficial bladder tumors (PR + CR = 65%) when applied in 12 one-hour daily treatments. When applied to invasive bladder cancer cases, topical hyperthermia had occasional marked tumor necrosis.[33] However, elevating the bladder temperature beyond 50C to provide deeper hyperthermic penetration led to severe toxicity.[36]

Other cavities that could be heated from the surface of the interior might include stomach, colon, peritoneal and pleural cavities. Spratt et al.[38] developed a system that delivered hyperthermic fluid to the peritoneal cavity at 45C but also raised the systemic temperature to 41C. Filter systems removed cells from being recirculated. A patient with pseudomyxoma peritonei was then treated with two courses for 1 1/2 hours at 42C IP temperature. Thiotepa and Methotrexate were added to the heated perfusion. The patient underwent a significant PR for at least eight months.[39] In a rat model of intraperitoneal hyperthermia, temperatures dropped 1C at 1 mm deep from the peritoneal surface but only .2C at 1 mm deep from the bowel serosa.[40] The small bowel tolerance to hyperthemia is thus the limiting factor to applying intraperitoneal hyperthermia. The most sensitive cells to hyperthermia are the gut luminal nonproliferative cells which can tolerate only 10-20 minutes at 43C.[41] No damaging effects are seen at 42C for one hour, however.

The application of heat to a surface presents many problems in the non-uniform distribution of the hyperthermia.[42] The vascularity of normal tissues and tumors will determine the temperatures achieved. The application of heat to one surface will produce a temperature gradient from the bath temperature to normothermia at a variable depth. Precise measurement of tumor temperature is difficult.[43] The geometry of the tumor (often partially unknown), variable vascularity, and imprecise methods of thermal probe placement make interpretation of temperatures difficult. Some human tumors are considered to seed along needle tracks, adding a risk to the use of needle thermistors.

INTRAVESICAL HYPERTHERMIA AND INTRA-ARTERIAL CHEMOTHERAPY

We have treated 16 patients in a phase I manner with a combination of local intravesical hyperthermia and IA chemotherapy. All patients had bulky pelvic clinical stage C bladder cancer. The diagnosis of invasive bladder cancer was established by transurethral biopsy and showed deep muscle invasion with grade II-IV transitional cell carcinoma. These biopsies served as control tissues, and no biopsy displayed any tissue necrosis. Staging evaluation included bimanual examination under anesthesia, excretory urography, computerized tomography scan of the abdomen, chest tomography, bone scan, liver/spleen scan, and liver function tests.

Via a percutaneous femoral artery route, bilateral arterial catheters were placed just distal to the origin of the superior gluteal artery. The chemotherapeutic agent, ADR or CDDP, was infused with a Harvard pump over 48 hours. Patients were hydrated in the standard manner if they received CDDP.

Local bladder hyperthermia was achieved by pump circulation of heated water through a 24 Fr three-way urethral catheter. Inflow and outflow temperatures were continuously monitored with thermistors. The outflow temperature was escalated through our series, and we now use 45C. This level can be maintained safely for 96 hours and requires a 47-49C inflow temperature. Outflow resistance was adjusted so as to maintain the bladder in an approximately half-filled state (200 cc).

Cystoscopy was performed every 7-10 days to evaluate the bladder luminal surface. Serum creatinine, WBC count, and platelet count were monitored every 1-3 days. At 4 weeks the patients underwent exploratory laparotomy and radical cystoprostatectomy if metastatic disease was not present outside the pelvis. Only two of the 16 patients did not undergo resections of their cancers.

INTRA-ARTERIAL ADRIAMYCIN PLUS INTRAVESICAL HYPERTHERMIA

Our first group of nine patients received 40-75 mg/m^2 IA ADR over 48 hours with the dose escalating after every third patient.[44] Bladder hyperthermia was maintained for the 48 hours of infusion plus 48 hours post-infusion. The temperature was escalated over the series from 39C to 45C.

Clinically the patients tolerated the protocol extremely well. Leukopenia occurred in two patients, and the bladder hyperthermia caused only mild bladder discomfort relieved by anticolinergics. Though the regimen caused significant tumor necrosis, only one cystectomy specimen was NED. Seven of the nine patients died 9-220 weeks (mean equals 60 weeks) postoperatively of metastatic bladder cancer. The other two patients died 12 and 22 weeks postoperatively of unrelated causes.

The tumor necrosis seen pathologically was clearly a gradient from bladder luminal surface to bladder serosal surface. We could not prove any synergism occuring between the ADR and hyperthermia. At this time, Hahn suggested that hyperthermia may cause a heat-induced tolerance by cells to exposure to ADR and that synergism may not work in clinical therapy.[24] CDDP appeared to be the most effective single agent against bladder cancer and to be synergistic with hyperthermia in tumor model systems.[28]

INTRA-ARTERIAL CDDP PLUS INTRAVESICAL HYPERTHERMIA

Seven male patients have undergone hypogastric artery infusion of CDDP over 48 hours with concomitant local bladder hyperthermia. The bladder temperature was 45C, and the CDDP dose was escalated after every third patient from 100 mg/m^2 to 125 mg/m^2. Complications of the preoperative CDDP and hyperthermia were minimal. One patient had bladder spasms, which were treated with anticholinergics, and one patient developed an asymptomatic urinary tract infection. Myelosuppression was not seen, and no serum creatinine rose more than 2.2 mg%. All creatinines promptly returned to pretreatment levels. During the CDDP infusion, patients developed only very minimal nausea, which was easily controlled with Compazine. This finding could be due to the slowness of our infusion, or possibly the IA route causes less nausea.

After four weeks, all patients were explored surgically, and five radical cystoprostatectomies were able to be performed. The cancers were bulky and seven ureters were obstructed. Two patients required hemodialysis and percutaneous nephrostomy before the protocol could begin.

Table 3: Clinical data on CDDP patients

Pt	Age	Tumor Grade	Pathologic State	Operation	Survival
1	63	IV	D	Exploratory laparotomy	d.11 wks TCC
2	56	II	C	Radical cystectomy	124 wks NED
3	61	III	C	Radical cystectomy	120 wks NED
4	62	III	C	Radical cystectomy	d.42 wks TCC
5	55	III	D	Exploratory laparotomy	100 wks TCC persistent
6	64	III	D	Radical cystectomy	d.20 wks TCC
7	58	IV	D	Radical cystectomy	60 wks NED

PATHOLOGIC EFFECTS OF CDDP/HYPERTHERMIA

The tumor necrosis seen in the patients receiving IA CDDP plus bladder hyperthermia tended again to be somewhat in a gradient from the luminal surface to the serosal surface in four of the seven patients. However, in three of the seven patients necrosis of all invasive cancer was seen.

Table 4: Pathologic findings post cystectomy

	Primary Tumor Necrosis				Uninvolved Bladder			
Pt	Luminal surface tumor	Detrusor tumor	Peri-vesical tumor	Metastasis	Urothelium	Submucosa	Detrusor	Peri-vesica fat
1	NA	+	0	lymph nodes liver	NA	NA	NL	NL
2	4+	4+	4+		NL	edema	NL	NL
3	4+	2+	0		NL	edema	NL	NL
4	4+	4+	4+		NL	edema	NL	NL
5	3+	+	0	lymph nodes liver	NA	NA	NA	NL
6	+	0	0	lymph nodes	NL	edema	NL	NL
7	3+	4+	4+		NL	edema		NL

0 = no necrosis, tumor unchanged from previous biopsy
+ = < 25% residual tumor necrotic
2+ = 50% residual tumor necrotic
3+ = 75% residual tumor necrotic
4+ = 100% residual tumor necrotic
NA = not available
NL = normal

The normal urothelial surface was minimally affected by the treatment. The five cystectomy specimens that had histological examination of non-tumor areas showed only some minimal flattening of the intact transitional epithelium. The submucosa in non-tumor areas of the five bladders did show edema and venous dilatation to a moderate degree. The detrusor muscle bundles were not affected by the treatment. Perivesical fat in all seven patients was histologically normal in areas uninvolved by tumor. These histologic findings are in agreement with those of Meshorer et al.[(45)], who found 46-48C was required to produce significant necrosis in muscle and adipose tissue.

In the areas of tumor involvement, six bladder specimens had full thickness tumor available for histologic study. In all six, luminal surface tumor necrosis was present. Luminal surface necrosis was also seen cystoscopically in the seventh patient, but no tissue was obtained. One patient had some benign grade I papillary residual tumor on the surface, but all grade IV invasive tumor was necrotic. The tumor surfaces displayed coagulation necrosis with a mild neutrophilic infiltrate. Deep to this was a zone of nonviable tumor with fibrosis and ghosts of tumor cells. Deeper still was an area of tumor cells reacting to injury. Cell membranes were undefineable and frequently tumor cells coalesced into giant cells. The cytoplasm was either vacuolized or became densely eosinophillic. The nuclei were enlarged. In four of the seven bladders, tumor was still present within the detrusor muscle. The serosal surfaces of all bladders were available for study, and four of these had viable tumor present perivesically.

The ureters and prostate glands from the cystectomy specimens showed no effects of the treatment. Pelvic lymph nodes were examined in all seven patients, and these were reactive in four patients and contained metastatic tumor in three patients. Two patients had transitional cell carcinoma in the liver, and one patient had an incidental separate hepatocellular carcinoma. No tumor necrosis was seen in the metastases in lymph nodes or liver.

PLATINUM DISTRIBUTION

Patient 4 had total venous plasma platinum concentration measured immediately on completion of his 48 hour CDDP infusion, and this was 2.96 ug/ml (or approximately 10% of the administered dose still in the plasma). This is in line with the recently published levels of 2.71 ± .87 ug/ml[6] reported for hypogastric artery infusions of 60-120 mg CDDP over a median duration of infusion of 11.8 hours in 10 patients reported by Stewart et al.[(6)] Tissue platinum levels were measured by flameless atomic absorption spectroscopy. Results were expressed as ppm (ug platinum/gram of tissue) and are accurate to ± .05 ppm. Table 5 shows tissue platinum levels on specimens obtained at the time of surgical exploration.

Table 5: Tissue Platinum Levels (ug/g tissue).

Patient	Luminal tumor	1 cm deep tumor	Univolved Mucosa	Detrusor	Perivesical Fat	Prostate
3	<1.5				<.51	
4	3.8	6.4		1.2		.5
5		<1.6			<.41	
6	1.1	.83	.82	.69	<.56	.91
7	1.2	1.0			<.8	4.5

It is difficult to know what tissue platinum values actually mean. Few values have been reported for human tumors treated clinically. Bonnem et al.[(46)] reported a platinum level of 1.6 ppm in a glioblastoma treated with five courses of 60 mg/m^2 CDDP. Jaffe et al.[(12)] reported on platinum levels in osteosarcoma and in uninvolved bone in eight patients who had undergone 2-4 IA infusions for osteosarcoma. Their data is reported in ug/g dry weight which makes it difficult to compare. They showed that those tumors with the greatest concentrations of platinum also showed the greatest tumor destruction. In our data, patients 4 and 6 are the most interesting. Patient 4 had a bulky grade III transitional cell carcinoma that was completely destroyed by the IA CDDP/bladder hyperthermia treatment. His tumor markedly concentrated platinum compared to his uninvolved bladder detrusor muscle. The patient died of distant metastatic transitional cell carcinoma, showing the spillover CDDP did not eradicate his distant disease. Patient 6 had a signet cell carcinoma of the bladder with an elevated serum CEA of 130 ng/ml (normal < 3.1 ng/ml). Histologically, very little effect was seen due to the CDDP/hyperthermia pretreatment. Platinum levels in his tumor tissue were not different from levels in uninvolved bladder. The patient died rapidly from abdominal and pelvic metastases.

Other tissues found to have low detectable platinum values included pelvic lymph nodes (.35-.5 ppm), rectus muscle, ileum, and subcutaneous fat. Liver biopsies in two patients showed .62 and .83 ppm. This represents retention of approximately 3% of the administered dose in the liver. This is in agreement with animal studies showing significant liver retention of IV administered CDDP.[47]

It appears from our series that IA CDDP/local bladder hyperthermia is safe and has minimal side effects. The CDDP dose can be escalated further. While our method of intracavitary hyperthermia application has the advantage of being able to be much prolonged compared to other modalities of hyperthermia, the tumor temperatures achieved must clearly be nonuniform. In our next phase of the study, needle thermistors are being placed in the tumors to characterize the thermal gradient. Bladder cancer tumor necrosis has been seen with our protocol but varies considerably between tumors. The delivery of IA CDDP can cause significant uptake of CDDP into the cancer, as evidenced by the 5.4-fold increase in bladder cancer platinum uptake compared to uninvolved bladder muscle seen in patient 4. Long-term retention of platinum by the liver is also seen. Systemic spillover of the CDDP does occur, but no evidence of systemic anti-tumor effect was observed.

REFERENCES

1. Swistel AJ, Hancock CH, Bading JR, Leyland-Jones B, Raaf JH: Pharmacokinetics of Intra-arterial versus intravenous Adriamycin in the VX-2 tumor system. Surgical forum 34:443-444, 1983.
2. Didolkar MS, Kanter PM, Baffi RR, Schwartz HS, Lopez R, Baez N: Comparison of regional versus systemic chemotherapy with Adriamycin. Ann Surg (187):332-336, 1978.
3. Kraybill WG, Harrison M, Sasaki T, Fletcher WS: Regional intra-arterial infusion of Adriamycin in the treatment of cancer. Surg Gynec & Obstet (144):335-338, 1977.
4. Nakazono M, Iwata S: Intra-arterial infusion as a preoperative chemotherapeutic treatment for bladder tumor. American Urological Association annual meeting, San Francisco, California, May 18-22, 1980.
5. Benjamin R.S., Riggs C.E., Jr., Bachur N.R.: Pharmacokinetics and metabolism of Adriamycin in man. Clin Pharmacol Ther (14):592-600, 1973.
6. Stewart DJ, Benjamin RS, Zimmerman S, Caprioli RM, Wallace S, Chuang V, Calvo D III, Samuels M, Bonura J, Loo TL: Clinical Pharmacology of intra-arterial cis-diamminedicloroplatinum (II). Cancer Res (43):917-920,1983.
7. Carlson JA, Freedman RS, Wallace S, Chuang VP, Wharton JT, Rutledge FN: Intra-arterial cis-platinum in the management of squamous cell carcinoma of the uterine cervix. Gynecol Oncol (12):92-98, 1981.
8. Cheng E, Watson RC, Fortner J, Kemeny N, Golbey R: Regional intra-arterial infusion of cisplatin in primary liver cancer: A phase II trial. Proc Am Soc Clin Oncol (1):179, 1982.
9. Baker S, Wheeler R, Meduec B, Keller J, Keyes J, Ensminger W: Out-patient intra-arterial chemotherapy in head and neck cancer patients using a totally implanted infusion system. Proc Am Soc Clin Oncol (11):195, 1982.
10. Horiuchi M, Inuyama Y, Kohno N: Clinical pharmacology of intra-arterial and intravenous cis-diamminedichloroplatinum (II). Proc XIII International Cancer Congress 13:60, 1982.
11. Ajani JA, Burgess MA: Multiple squamous cell carcinoma treated with intra-arterial cisplatin in a patient with rheumatoid arthritis. Cancer Treatment Reports (66):1987-1989, 1982.
12. Jaffe N, Knapp J, Chuang VP, Wallace S, Ayala A, Murray J, Cangir A, Wang A, Benjamin RS: Osteosarcoma: Intra-arterial treatment of the primary tumor with cis-diammine-dichloroplatinum II (CDP). Cancer (51):402-407, 1983.
13. Calvo DB III, Patt YZ, Wallace S, Chuang VP, Benjamin RS, Pritchard JD, Hersh EM, Bodey GP Sr, Mavligit GM: Phase I-II trial of intra-arterial cis-diammine dichloroplatinum (II) for regionally confined malignancy. Cancer (45):1278-1283, 1980.
14. Stewart DJ, Wallace S, Feun L, Leavens M, Young SE, Handel S, Mavligit G, Benjamin RS: A Phase I study of intracarotid artery infusion of cis-diammine dichloroplatinum (II) in patients with recurrent malignant intracerebral tumors. Cancer Research (42):2059-2062, 1982.
15. Pritchard JD, Mavligit GM, Benjamin RS, Patt YZ, Calvo DB, Hall SW, Bodby GP, Wallace S: Regression of regionally confined melanoma with intra-arterial cis-dichlorodiammine platinum (II). Cancer Treatment Rep 63.

16. Wallace S, Chuang VP, Samuels M, Johnson D: Transcatheter Intra-arterial infusion of chemotherapy in advanced bladder cancer. Cancer (49):640-645, 1982.
17. Dewey WC, Saparetto SA, Betten DA: Hyperthermic radiosensitization of synchronous Chinese hamster cells and relation between lethality and chromosomal aberrations. Radiation Res (76): 48-59, 1978.
18. Gerner EW: Thermotolerance in hyperthermia in cancer therapy. In Storm FK (ed) GK Hall, Boston, 1983, pp 141-162.
19. Song CW: Blood flow in tumors and normal tissues in hyperthermia in cancer therapy. In: Storm FK (ed) GK Hall, Boston, 1983, pp 187-206.
20. Herman TS, Baustian AM, Kundrat MA: Enhancement of hyperthermia induced lethality and modulation of Adriamycin cytotoxicity by cooling. Proc Am Assoc Can Res (22):221, 1981.
21. Vig BK: Effect of hypothermia and hyperthermia on the induction of chromosome aberrations by Adriamycin in human leukocytes. Cancer Res (38):550-555, 1978.
22. Hahn GM, Braun J, Har-Kedar I: Thermochemotherapy: Synergism between hyperthermia (42-43° C) and adriamycin (or bleomycin) in mammalian cell inactivation. Proc Natl Acad Sci USA (72):937:940, 1975.
23. Marmor JB: Interactions of hyperthermia and chemotherapy in animals. Cancer Res (39):2269-2276, 1979.
24. Hahn GM: Potential for therapy of drugs and hyperthermia. Cancer Res (39):2264-2268, 1979.
25. Meyn RE, Corry PM, Fletcher SE, Demetriades M: Thermal enhancement of DNA damage for mammalian cells treated with cis-diamminedichloro-platinum (II). Cancer Res (40):1136-1139, 1980.
26. Fisher GA, Hahn GM: Enhancement of cis-platinum (II) diammine-dichloride cytotoxicity by hyperthermia. Natl Cancer Inst Monogram (61):255-257, 1982.
27. Brouwer J, Fichtinger-Schepman AMJ, Van de Putte P, and Reedijk J: Influence of temperature on platinum binding to DNA, cell killing, and mutation induction in escherichia coli K-12 cells treated with cis-diamminedichloroplatinum (II). Cancer Res (42):2416-2419, 1982.
28. Alberts DS, Peng YM, Chen HSG, Moon TE, Cetas TL, and Hoeschele JD: Therapeutic synergism of hyperthermia-cis-platinum in a mouse tumor model. J.N.C.I. (65):455-461, 1980.
29. Quebbman EJ, Skibba JL, Petroff RJ Jr: A technique for isoated hyperthermic liver perfusion. J Surg Oncol (in press).
30. Cavaliere R, Mondovi B, Moricca G, Monticelli G, Natali PG, Santori FS, DiFillippo F, Varenese A, Aloe L, Rossi-fanelli A: Regional perfusion hyperthermia. In: Storm FK (ed) Hyperthermia in cancer therapy. GK Hall, Boston, 1983, pp 369-399.
31. Hild P, Aigner K, Henneking K: Levels of cis-platinum in hyperthermic isolated perfusion. Anticancer Res (2):225-256, 1982.
32. Hall RR, Schade ROK, Swinney J: Effects of hyperthermia on bladder cancer. Br J Urol (2):593-594, 1974.
33. England HR, Anderson JD, Minasian H, Marshall VR, Molland EA, Blandy JP: The therapeutic application of hyperthermia in the bladder. Br J Urol (47):849-851, 1975.
34. Rege VB, Leone LA, Soderberg CH Jr, Coleman GV, Robidoux HJ, Fijman R, Brown J: Hyperthermic adjuvant perfusion chemotherapy for stage I malignant melanoma of the extremity with literature review. Cancer (52):2033-2039, 1983.

35. Wile A, Juler GL, Rosenberg H, Haiouc N, Stemmer EA: Control of pelvic cancer with hyperthermic isolation-perfusion. J Surg Res (34):560-567, 1983.
36. Hall RR, Wadehra V, Towler JR, Hindmarsh JR, Byrne PO: Hyperthermia in the treatment of bladder tumours. Br J Urol (48):603-608, 1976.
37. Shingelton WW, Parker RT, Mahaley S: Abdominal perfusion for cancer chemotherapy with hypothermia and hyperthermia. Surgery (50):260-265, 1961.
38. Spratt JS, Adcock RA, Sherrill W, Travathon S: Hyperthermic peritoneal perfusion system in canines. Cancer Res (40):253-255, 1980.
39. Spratt JS, Adcock RA, Muskovin M, Sherrill W, McKeown J: Clinical delivery system for intraperitoneal hyperthermic chemotherapy. Cancer Res (40):256:260, 1980.
40. Shiu MH, Fortner JG: Intraperitoneal hyperthermic treatment of implanted peritoneal cancer in rats. Cancer Res (40):4081-4084, 1980.
41. Hume SP, Marigold JCL, Michalowski A: The effect of local hyperthermia on nonproliferative, compared with proliferative, epithelial cells of mouse intestinal mucosa. Radiat Res (94)252-262, 1983.
42. Jain RK: Bioheat transfer: Mathematical models of thermal systems. In: Storm FK (ed) Hyperthermia in cancer therapy. GK Hall, Boston, 1983, pp 9-46.
43. Christensen DA: Thermometry and thermography. In: Storm FK (ed). Hyperthermia in cancer therapy. GK Hall, Boston, 1983, pp 223-232.
44. Jacobs SC, Lawson RK: Pathologic effects of pre-cystectomy therapy with combination intra-arterial doxorubicin hydrochloride and local bladder hyperthermia for bladder cancer. J Urol (127):43-47, 1982.
45. Meshorer A, Prionas SD, Fajardo, LF, Meyer JL, Hahn GM, Martinez AA: The effects of hyperthermia on normal mesenchymal tissues. Arch Pathol Lab Med (107)328-334, 1983.
46. Bonnem EM, Litterst CL, Smith FP: Platinum concentrations in human glioblastoma multiforme following the use of cisplatin. Cancer Treat Rep (66):1661-1663, 1983.
47. Litterst CL, LeRoy AF, Guarrino AM: Disposition and distribution of platinum following parenteral administration of cis-dichlorodiammine platinum (II) to animals. Cancer Treat Rep (63):1485-1492, 1979.

COMBINATION HYPERTHERMIA AND INTRA-ARTERIAL CHEMOTHERAPY

F.K. STORM, M.D.

MODERN CONCEPTS OF LOW-TEMPERATURE HYPERTHERMIA

Selective Thermosensitivity of Cancer Cells

At temperatures between 41°-45 C (106-113°F), cancer cells are slightly more sensitive to heat than their normal cell counterparts. In vitro and in vivo tumor models have shown irreversible damage and complete regression of various tumors at 42-45°C, while normal cells were killed at at least one degree higher temperature or more than double the duration of heating.

Mechanism of Action

Hyperthermia causes alteration in both DNA and RNA synthesis, as well as depression of multiple cellular enzymatic systems required for cell metabolism and division. Its major mode of action may be to increase cell and lysosome membrane permeability, causing selective internal destruction of the cancer cell. Less-well-oxygenated cells seem to be most vulnerable to thermic injury.

Histologic Tissue Alteration

Heat causes progressive necrosis of tumor cells at these temperatures but not in stromal or vascular cells within tumors nor in normal surrounding tissues. Autolytic disintegration of heat-damaged cells is followed by a marked increase in connective tissue stroma and scar formation.

Interestingly, this occurs in tissue cultures of tumor-derived and tumor-producing cells, but not in normal and non-tumor-producing cells. When a cell subline derived from a non-tumor-producing line acquires high tumor-producing ability, it also acquires greater thermosensitivity. Thus, the acquisition of malignant potential, both in vivo and in vitro, is accompanied by decreased thermotolerance.

THERMO CHEMOTHERAPY

In 1973, Johnson and Pavelec reported that the tumoricidal effects of thiotepa (5μg/ml) on V-79 Chinese hamster cells were enhanced times 2-logs by elevating temperatures from 37°C to 42°C. That year, Muckle and Dickson reported that 43°C hyperthermia combined with methotrexate at dosages of 0.4mg/kg had more than double the effectiveness of drug alone on VX2 tumors in rabbits. In 1975, Hahn et al. found that an increase in temperature to 43°C would enhance the cell kill of doxorubicin (and bleomycin) by 3 logs in the EMT-6 sarcoma model compared with normothermic (37°C) temperatures. Equally interesting, they observed that doxorubicin, usually unable to cross the membrane into the EMT-6 sarcoma cell, crossed the cell membrane under hyperthermic conditions. These observations supported the postulate that heat alters cell membrane permeability.[13,14.] Should this phenomenon occur in humans, substantial preferential tumor kill might take place.

In the treatment of locally recurrent and intransit melanoma of the extremities using hyperthermic limb perfusion, Stehlin found an increased response from 35% to 80% by the addition of heat (41°C) to melphalan perfusion.

Recent determinations[27]by the clonogenic human stem cell assay performed by our group at normothermic (37°C) and at hyperthermic (42°C) temperatures suggest that hyperthermia may significantly enhance tumor kill over drug alone.

Since we have found that intraarterial drug infusion therapy is superior to the i.v. route for some primary and secondary liver cancers, the potential ability of heat to enhance intracellular drug concentration might increase clinical response. These contentions have led to combined-therapy clinical trials of intraarterial hepatic chemotherapy and hyperthermia at our institution.

HYPERTHERMIA TECHNIQUE

The majority of clinical trials of visceral hyperthermia

have been conducted with the radiofrequency magnetic loop induction system called the Magnetrode™. Fortunately, magnetic loop applicators can effectively heat a large region of the body (thorax or abdomen). Since the exact location of all boundaries and extensions of a tumor need not be known, this device has proved to be very useful for evaluating the effects of deep hyperthermia of cancers invading one or several adjacent visceral organs, especially liver.

CLINICAL TRIALS

Melanoma

Ten consecutive patients with documented melanoma metastases to the liver and an absence of brain metastases were treated with IA-DTIC and hyperthermia at temperatures of 40.8-41.5°C, and eight achieved disease regression or stabilization from 3 to 14 mo (6.5 mo median). There was one complete response for 11 mo, two partial responses for 7 and 14 mo, one minimal response for 3 mo, and four patients had no progression in their disease associated with stabilization or improvement in physical status for 3, 3, 6, and 7.5 months. Seven patients retained or regained a normal activity status, and 4/5 patients with significant liver pain experienced complete pain relief subsequent to treatment. Seven patients died at 3-18 months (8.5 month median). All therapy responders died of brain metastases. Liver disease only progressed during the latter phases of their illnesses.

Colon Carcinoma

Because of the poor prognosis for patients with liver metastases from colon carcinoma who are treated with conventional intravenous 5-FU, the UCLA Division of Surgical Oncology devised a unique therapy plan consisting of distal hepatic artery ligation followed by continuous infusion of 5-FU through the proximal hepatic artery and monthly hyperthermia treatment. The rationale for the therapy plan was based on several recent findings. Because liver metastases generally receive their blood supply from the hepatic artery, interruption of the arterial flow alone could cause some degree of tumor necrosis. Moreover, since effective hyperthermia of many solid tumors appears to be highly dependent on a reduced tumor blood flow, interruption of the arterial supply could further impair the tumor's ability to dissipate heat and induce increased independent tumor temperatures. Direct infusion of the chemotherapy also could increase the extracellular drug gradient at the site of the tumor with less systemic drug toxicity. Hyperthermia appears to be tumoricidal as a single agent but might also increase intracellular uptake of drug in the target tissue.

A prospective randomized trial is now underway to evaluate combined thermochemotherapy for colon metastases in liver. The role of hepatic artery ligation and infusion therapy is being compared with conventional i.v. 5-FU administration. Of 11 patients initially treated with 5-FU and hepatic hyperthermia, one had complete response at 13 months follow-up, one had partial response at 9 months, and seven patients had no progression of disease at 3-8 months (5 months median).

REFERENCES

1. Storm FK, Harrison WH, Morton DL, et al: Human hyperthermia therapy. Relationship between tumor type and capacity to induce hyperthermia by radiofrequency. Am J Surg 138:170-174, 1979.
2. Storm FK, Harrison WH, Morton DL, et al: Normal tissue and solid tumor effects of hyperthermia in animal models and clinical trials. Cancer Res 39:2245-2251, 1979.
3. Storm FK, Elliott RS, Harrison WH, et al: Hyperthermia therapy for human neoplasms. Thermal death time. Cancer 46:1849-1854, 1980
4. Mann BD. Storm FK, Kern DH, Giuliano A, Morton DL: Predictive value of the clonogenic assay in the treatment of melanoma with DTIC and DTIC + hyperthermia. Proc Am Soc Clin Oncol 17:432, 1981.
5. Storm FK, Morton DL: Hyperthermia: Adjunctive modality for hepatic infusion chemotherapy. Sem in Oncol 10:223-227, 1983.
6. Storm FK, Kaiser LR, Goodnight JE, et al: Thermochemotherapy for melanoma metastases in liver. Cancer 49:1243-1248, 1982.
7. Storm FK (ed): Hyperthermia in Cancer Therapy. Boston, GK Hall Medical Publishers, 1983.